DISCOVER **THE SPEAK METHOD**

FEEL YOUTHFUL AT ANY AGE

Be Younger Next Month

KATHY ANNE JONES

Copyright © 2024 by Kathryn Jones

All rights are reserved, and no part of this publication may be reproduced, distributed, or transmitted in any manner, whether through photocopying, recording, or any other electronic or mechanical methods, without the explicit prior written permission of the publisher. This restriction applies to any form or means of reproduction or distribution.

Exceptions to this rule include brief quotations that may be incorporated into critical reviews, as well as certain other noncommercial uses that are allowed by copyright law. Any such usage must adhere to the specified conditions and permissions outlined by the copyright holder.

Book Design by HMDPUBLISHING

Dedication

To my younger sister Anne, who has faced and overcome countless challenges throughout her life.

Your strength and unwavering spirit are a beautiful reflection of Mom's kindness and sweet nature. I'll always remember your love of animals, even the stuffed ones. Anne, you inspire me every day, and my heart is filled with gratitude to have you as my sister.

Love you always and forever.

In Gratitude

I could fill an entire book with my gratitude for those who have supported me throughout my life's journey and now as an author, but here goes.

- First, my mother and father, for instilling in me the values that I continue to uphold today.
- My husband, Harvey, who was my biggest supporter and took over the household chores while I shut myself in the office to write.
- My stepdaughter, Brooke, whom I affectionately call my special daughter, tirelessly editing, proofreading, and continually encouraging me.
- My friend, Lynda, intuitively knowing it was the perfect time to reconnect after so many years.
- Bridget and John, owners of The Health Dare, for giving me the opportunity to change thousands of lives over the last 7 ½ years, I am forever grateful.
- My forever-young friend, Cody, whose laughter and inspiration have always reminded me to never give up.
- All my siblings, nieces, and nephews, for supporting "Crazy Aunt Kathy" in her pursuit of a natural lifestyle, fully aware that visits to my home would be filled with the fragrance of essential oils and the aroma of new foods.

Introducing The SPEAK Method

Confucius wisely said, *"Life is really simple, but we insist on making it complicated."*

Are you feeling overwhelmed by the abundance of advice on aging gracefully and joyfully? Life was simpler before the internet and social media, when we relied on the wisdom of our parents, grandparents, teachers, and neighbors for guidance.

Be Younger Next Month clears the confusion! With over four decades of experience as a natural chef and wellness expert, I am thrilled to present **The SPEAK Method**—a straightforward yet effective framework featuring 30 days of enjoyable activities to help you feel youthful at any age.

SPEAK is an acronym I have crafted to represent the foundational pillars to unlock your youthful potential.

Selfcare: Practice It Daily

Passion: Discover and Ignite It

Eat and Enjoy: Nourishing Food

Activity: Embrace and Love Movement

Kindness: Cultivate it in Your Daily Life

Discover over 150 insights to effortlessly weave these principles into your daily routine, ensuring a lasting and positive transformation.

Listen to heartfelt interviews with doctors, experts, moms, and everyday people who have embraced this approach to feel youthful at any age.

Each chapter includes a journal section to track your daily activities and experiences.

Enjoy 30 days of healthy, delicious recipes inspired by my organic restaurant, natural foods store deli, and personal chef services. These recipes will delight your taste buds while nourishing your body, making your journey to a younger you enjoyable and sustainable.

Let's explore the fundamentals of The SPEAK Method!

SELF-CARE – PRACTICE IT DAILY

Legendary childhood actress Lucille Ball humorously remarked, *"Love yourself first, and everything else falls into line. You really have to love yourself to get anything done in this world."*

Embarking on a journey to feel younger starts with embracing self-care and self-love, no matter your life stage. Contrary to popular belief, self-love is not egotistical; it is an expression of self-appreciation.

One of my cherished self-care rituals is indulging in massages. My brother and his Thai wife introduced me to Thailand, aptly named, "The Land of Smiles". During my delightful stay, I enjoyed daily massages, sometimes two a day, as they were surprisingly affordable at just $5 - $10 per hour. I highly recommend adding 'Massage in Thailand' to your bucket list.

If you're not planning a trip to Thailand or another dream destination, consider treating yourself to a massage, indulging in a facial, or relaxing with your favorite book or movie—each a wonderful form of self-care.

Remember, the foundation of caring for and loving others rests on your ability to prioritize and care for yourself first. As echoed in the movie "The Help," affirm to yourself: *"You are smart, you are kind, you are important."*

Inside, you will find valuable guidance and insights to help you embrace self-love and practice self-care. Treat yourself with the kindness and love you deserve because you are worth it!

PASSION – DISCOVER AND IGNITE IT

Renowned author Wayne Dyer once advised, *"Don't die with your music still in you!"* Your unique "music" is your passion. What ignites your enthusiasm and brings you joy?

My journey began at a young age, discovering a love for cooking under my mother's loving guidance. Growing up in the Midwest, known for its meat and exceptionally sweet corn, my culinary world expanded when my Massachusetts grandfather introduced our family to fresh lobsters. Despite the initial shock of immersing them into boiling water—a moment where I mistakenly perceived their silent descent as screams—their sweet taste captivated me.

My passion for cooking inspired me to open Iowa's first organic restaurant, where I catered for distinguished figures such as President Gerald Ford, the Neville Brothers, and the Joffrey Ballet. My love for skiing led my husband and me to Colorado, where we owned a natural foods store and deli. Our adventures continued in Panama, living on an organic coffee farm and immersing ourselves in the culture and flavors of the local cuisine.

Now, I reside in the scenic mountains of North Carolina, dedicating my time to health coaching, teaching cooking classes, personal cheffing, and natural product development. This journey has allowed me to share my passion for nourishing whole foods in meaningful ways.

You will find guidance to identify your passions and incorporate them into your daily life. Discovering your passions is a journey, but the pursuit is always worth it to find what truly sparks your soul.

EAT AND ENJOY – NOURISHING FOOD

One of the first influential books I read on healthy eating was "Let's Eat Right to Keep Fit" by Adele Davis, published in 1954. It significantly promoted the importance of eating nourishing food. While the phrase *"You Are What You Eat"* may not solely be attributed to her, it reflects her teachings, which have guided me for most of my adult life.

Growing up, I faced weight issues, especially in a society that idealized figures like Twiggy. Being labeled as "chubby" made the journey harder. The prevalence of fad diets led to unconventional food choices, including a college staple of Velveeta cheese, canned green beans, and saltines. This experience led me to question diets—after all, what are the first three letters of "DIET"? Die! Diets aren't the solution; cultivating a healthy lifestyle is.

College became a turning point when my mother died of colon cancer, and my father faced cardiovascular issues. I am grateful to them for sparking my curiosity about the diet-disease link. In the pre-Google era, I spent countless hours researching this connection in the college library.

The granola era solidified my commitment to healthy eating. I adopted the mantra, *"If God made it, eat it. If man made it, don't eat it—or eat it in moderation."* Nature provides us with whole grains, vegetables, fruits, and proteins, while boxed mac and cheese is man-made. Which one are you choosing?

You are about to embark on a journey to enjoy nourishing food, while discovering insights and delectable recipes along the way.

ACTIVITY – EMBRACE AND LOVE MOVEMENT

Hippocrates, the Father of Modern Medicine, famously said, *"If you are in a bad mood, go for a walk. If you are still in a bad mood, go for another walk."*

Have you ever viewed exercise as a daunting eight-letter word? I certainly did! Gym classes were my nemesis, and being one of the last chosen for teams was disheartening.

Growing up in landlocked Iowa, our solace from hot afternoons was the local pool. Evenings were spent begging for more time in the water. Weekends meant trips to Clear Lake with friends and family, or the ocean near my grandparents' home in Massachusetts. Those beach days included swimming, running along the shore, and catching minnows for my grandfather, where I learned a valuable beach lesson: Never pick up a "balloon" on the beach, as my sister found out when she mistook a Portuguese Man of War for a balloon!

I've swum in lakes, rivers, and oceans across the US, Panama, Costa Rica, the Caribbean, Greece, Thailand, Hawaii, and beyond. Water is my element. By swapping exercise for physical activity or movement, I found joy and energy in activities that resonate with me. Whether it's a team sport, a walk in nature, a group class, a bike ride, or a swim—just move! As Nike's slogan says, "Just Do It!"

Discover simple movements that make your heart sing, and your body thrive, making movement an integral and delightful part of your daily routine.

KINDNESS – CULTIVATE IT IN YOUR DAILY LIFE

Maya Angelou, renowned author and poet, wisely said, *"People will forget what you said, people will forget what you did, but people will never forget how you made them feel."*

One of my cherished childhood memories is evening drives to an unexpected destination—the cemetery. With no air conditioning, we'd pile into the car, windows down, eagerly discussing the coveted front seat, and head to the countryside to escape the heat.

At the cemetery's lake, we coaxed the resident swans to shore with pieces of stale bread, sharing moments of admiration. Watching the elegant birds glide gracefully across the water brought a sense of peace and connection to nature. It felt like the swans recognized us each time we returned, their gentle approach and calm demeanor forming a unique bond.

As I grew older, I discovered that swans are incredibly intelligent and possess the ability to recognize and remember humans over long periods. If treated kindly, they tend to harbor positive feelings towards you. Swans also form lifelong partnerships, offering us profound lessons in loyalty and kindness. Their enduring commitment to one another and their gentle interactions remind us to treat others with compassion and respect.

Through these encounters, I came to understand the enduring impact of kindness in our relationships with people. The lessons learned from those graceful creatures continue to inspire me to approach life with a kind and open heart.

Discover how effortlessly you can weave daily acts of kindness into your day and help create a world overflowing with joy and contentment.

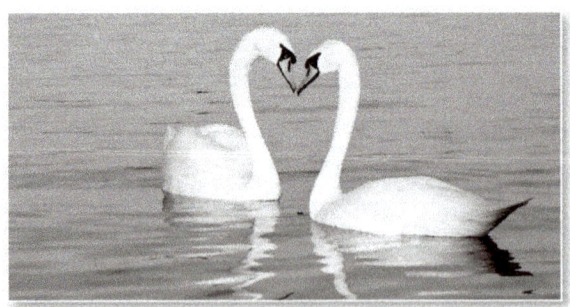

DAY 1

"Gratitude is not only the heart of happiness but the key to unlocking the fullness of life."
Brené Brown

SELF-CARE – PRACTICE IT DAILY

A simple way to start practicing self-care is by embracing gratitude. Appreciating the positive aspects of your life will foster a mindset of positivity and resilience. Twelve years ago, my husband suffered a severe bicycle accident that led to a brain injury. Upon his release from the hospital, he exhibited symptoms like those of a stroke victim. However, through good nutrition, prayer, the unwavering support of family and friends, and his stubborn Taurus trait, he pulled through and continues to ride his bike daily. It has not always been easy, but I am eternally grateful. Look for gratitude in your life.

Start a Gratitude Journal:

- Each morning, write down three things you're grateful for. They can be as simple as a warm cup of coffee, the feel of the morning sun on your skin, or the comforting presence of your pet. Embrace the significant things too, like strong family bonds and good health.

Practice Mindfulness:

- Find a quiet, comfortable space where you won't be disturbed. Close your eyes, take a few deep, slow breaths, and focus on the present moment, letting go of any worries. Appreciate the beauty around you, like the vibrant colors of a flower or the gentle rustling of leaves.

Be Specific:

- Make your expressions of gratitude more specific. Instead of general statements like "I'm grateful for my family," say, "I'm grateful for the laughter we shared at dinner." Being specific trains your mind to notice and cherish the finer details of everyday life.

This practice not only enhances your mood but also strengthens your resilience.

PASSION – DISCOVER AND IGNITE IT

Identify your passion by reflecting on childhood interests. Often, the activities we loved as children provide clues to our true passions as adults. In our youth, we engaged in activities purely out of love and curiosity, free from practical constraints or societal expectations.

Reconnect with Old Hobbies:

- Consider revisiting hobbies or interests you had as a child. If you love painting, try taking an art class and setting up a creative space at home. Re-engaging with these activities can reignite your passion and remind you of what you truly enjoy. Ask those who knew you well as a child what they remember you loved to do. Their insights can be very revealing.

Visualize Your Ideal Day as a Child:

- What activities would you engage in? This can help you tap into your authentic interests, offering a roadmap to activities that might still bring you joy. As a young child, my ideal day was spent at the beach with my grandparents watching Grandpa cook clams and lobster, sparking my passion for cooking.

Blend Past and Present:

- Consider how to integrate your childhood passions with your current skills and experiences. Were you fascinated by the natural world and enjoyed exploring the outdoors? You might find fulfillment in a career in environmental research or education. Did you dream of being a teacher, or writer? Start your first book or volunteer to help teach a class!

Reflecting on childhood dreams is a powerful exercise to uncover passions rooted in your authentic self.

EAT AND ENJOY – NOURISHING FOOD

Today, choose a food you love and make it healthy. Why not start with chocolate? As my beloved t-shirt from La France restaurant in Dillon, Colorado, says, "Life is uncertain, eat dessert first!" This playful reminder highlights the joy and spontaneity that dessert brings to our lives. Dark chocolate is a great choice for a healthy makeover due to its many health benefits.

Why and how to eat chocolate:

Rich in Antioxidants and Nutrients:

- Supports heart health by lowering blood pressure and can improve cholesterol. Its high flavonoid content helps reduce inflammation and protect cells from damage.

Supports Brain Health:

- Flavonoids in dark chocolate can also enhance cognitive function by increasing blood flow to the brain, improving attention, processing speed, and memory. Have brain fog, eat dark chocolate!

Make Chocolate Even Healthier:

- Choose pure cocoa powder or dark chocolate with at least 70%. Pure cocoa powder retains the natural benefits of cocoa beans without the added sugars and fats found in many commercial chocolates.

Incorporate Chocolate:

- Put cocoa powder in your morning coffee or in **Chocolate Almond Fat Bombs.**
- Add chocolate chips and nuts to popcorn for an afternoon snack.
- Melt chocolate with a little coconut oil to dip strawberries and bananas.
- Get adventurous and try a classic Mexican dish – Chicken Mole.

By selecting high-quality dark chocolate and being mindful of portions, you can indulge in one of life's pleasures.

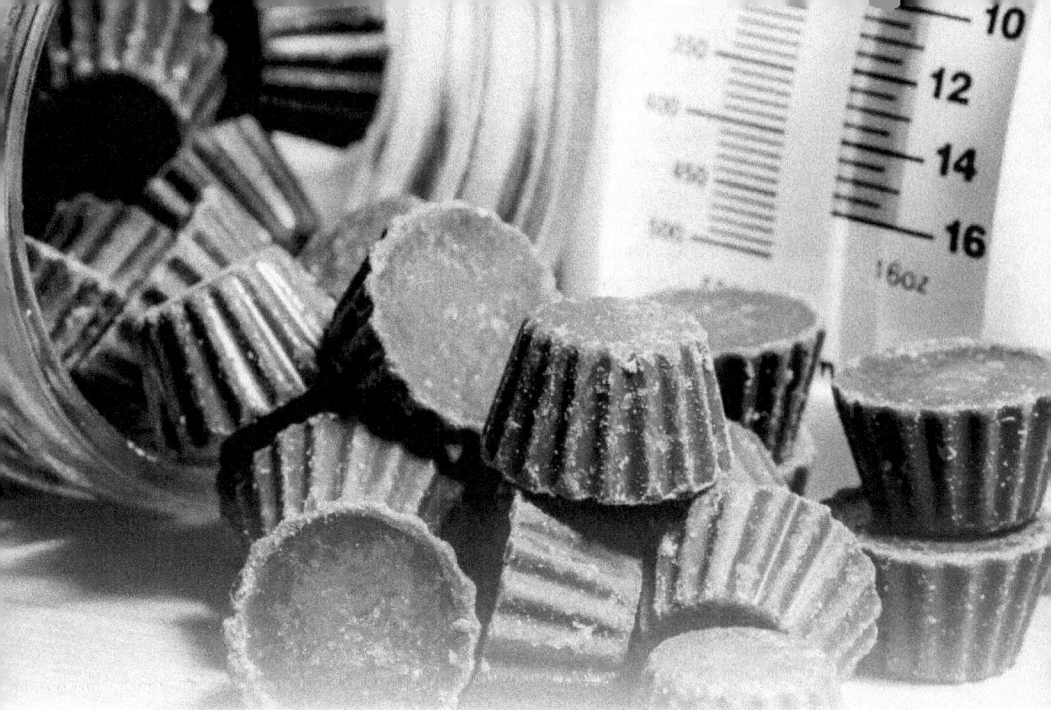

Chocolate Almond Fat Bombs

30 Servings

INGREDIENTS:

- ½ cup virgin coconut oil
- ½ cup sugar-free almond butter (can substitute peanut or any nut butter)
- 2-3 tablespoons unsweetened cocoa powder
- 2-4 tablespoons honey or pure maple syrup (sweeten to taste)
- 1/4 teaspoon vanilla extract
- Optional: Roasted sliced almonds and coarse sea salt

PROCESS:

1. In a small saucepan over low heat melt coconut oil and almond butter or other nut butter.
2. Stir in cocoa powder and honey. Remove from heat and add vanilla extract.

3. Pour into a spouted cup to make pouring easier and pour mixture into silicone candy molds. (Each mold should hold about 1 tablespoon of mixture)
4. Freeze or refrigerate until set. Remove from the molds and store in the refrigerator in an airtight container.
5. Alternative: If you do not have candy molds, use coconut oil to lightly oil a glass 8" x 8" baking dish. Pour mixture into dish and smooth with spatula. Refrigerate or freeze until set and cut into small squares.
6. Store in the refrigerator in an airtight container.
7. Optional: When chocolates are almost set, top with roasted sliced almonds or coarse sea salt.

ACTIVITY – EMBRACE AND LOVE MOVEMENT

When it comes to physical activity, why not make it fun? Hosting a dance party in your living room or dancing anywhere you please are excellent choices! So, crank up the music and unleash your moves on the "dance floor."

Move Freely:

- Don't worry about perfecting any dance moves or following a routine—just move your body in a way that feels good. Go ahead, dance like nobody's watching, and embrace the rhythm of life.

Heart Health Booster:

- Dancing is a great cardiovascular workout that improves your heart health, increases endurance, and can even help with co-ordination and balance. Plus, it releases endorphins, which are natural mood lifters. Feeling down, start dancing!

Build Connections:

- Invite your friends or family over for a dance party or make it a family event. Dancing together can strengthen relation-ships, create cherished memories, and encourage a sense of community.

Music Exploration:

- Dust off those old records, or find your favorite playlist, and let the music move you. Growing up near the Surf Ballroom in Clear Lake, Iowa, Buddy Holly's music was always playing in our home. One of my fondest teenage memories is dancing at the Surf. When I was 7 years old, his famous song "Peggy Sue" was released, and we jokingly thought it was written about my older sister Sue. Dancing to music that brings back memories can be incredibly uplifting.

Make dancing more and stressing less a priority in your life.

KINDNESS – CULTIVATE IT IN YOUR DAILY LIFE

Giving compliments is a wonderful way to cultivate kindness. By offering genuine, heartfelt compliments, we can uplift others and create a positive ripple effect in our communities. While I'm shopping, I make it a habit to start a conversation with someone by offering a simple compliment.

Be Genuine and Sincere:

- Look in the person's eyes, keep your arms relaxed, and use a friendly tone. Take the time to notice and appreciate the little things about those around you, whether it's a colleague's hard work, a friend's new haircut, or a stranger's smile. Be present in the moment; truly listen to what they are saying and respond with genuine interest and empathy.

Be Specific:

- Notice and appreciate an individual's unique qualities or efforts. Instead of generic compliments like, "You look great," be specific and personal. For instance, say, "I love your shoes! The color really suits you and adds a stylish touch to your outfit." Acknowledging details, like shoes, can make someone feel seen and valued. Similarly, "That is a cool shirt; you must be a Caitlin Clark, Iowa Hawkeye fan!" can spark conversation and create connections around sports teams.

Boost Your Mood:

- Compliments not only uplift the receiver but also have a positive effect on the giver. Practicing kindness through compliments can uplift your mood, and over time, this habit can create a ripple effect, inspiring others to spread kindness in their daily interactions.

*So, take a moment and start complimenting,
it can make the world a joyful place!*

Log Today's Activities and Experiences with The SPEAK Method

Use the questions or comments as a guide or write freely expressing your thoughts!

SELF-CARE – How did you practice Gratitude?

_____
_____
_____
_____
_____
_____
_____

PASSION – What childhood interests did you re-explore?

_____
_____
_____
_____
_____
_____
_____
_____

EAT AND ENJOY NOURISHING FOOD – Did you have some healthy chocolate or other sweets?

_____
_____
_____
_____
_____
_____
_____
_____

ACTIVITY – What songs did you dance to?

_____
_____
_____
_____
_____
_____
_____
_____

KINDNESS – Who did you compliment?

_____

_____

_____

_____

_____

ADDITIONAL NOTES

_____

_____

_____

_____

_____

DAILY REPORT CARD OF LIFE – How did you SPEAK today?

Grade Your Day, no D's or F's Allowed!

- **A** – Amazing
- **B** – Better than yesterday
- **C** – Challenging but working on it

DAY 2

> "So many things are possible as long as you don't know they are impossible."
> **Mildred D. Taylor**

SELF-CARE – PRACTICE IT DAILY

Caring for your skin, the body's largest organ, doesn't have to be overwhelming or costly. If you're short of time for a spa facial, try giving yourself one at home! Facials promote relaxation, boost circulation, and enhance your skin's appearance and health, leaving you feeling refreshed and pampered. Use ingredients in your kitchen with an easy-to-make, cost-effective solution that provides excellent results. Make it a relaxing ritual: light a candle and play some soothing music.

Egg White and Honey Facial Mask

INGREDIENTS:

- 1 egg white
- 1 teaspoon honey

PROCESS:

- Separate the egg white from the yolk (save the yolk for breakfast or another use).
- Whisk the egg white until it becomes foamy.
- Add the honey and mix well.
- Cleanse your face thoroughly and pat it dry.
- Using your fingers, apply the egg white mixture evenly to your face, avoiding the eye and mouth areas.
- Let the mask sit on your face for 15-20 minutes or until it dries completely.
- Gently rinse off the mask with lukewarm water and pat your face dry with a clean towel.
- Follow up with your favorite moisturizer to lock in hydration.

The egg white helps tighten your skin and shrink pores, while honey acts as a natural humectant, drawing moisture into your skin and keeping it hydrated. This combo will leave your skin feeling smooth, firm, and visibly refreshed.

Taking 15 minutes for yourself today can significantly impact how you feel and look, regardless of gender.

PASSION – DISCOVER AND IGNITE IT

Discovering your passion involves exploring new activities, hobbies, and experiences. By stepping out of your comfort zone and trying different pursuits, you open yourself to numerous possibilities.

Avoid Fear of Failure:

- Embrace a beginner's mindset and stay curious. Whether you're joining a dance class, experimenting with painting, or learning a musical instrument, each activity offers a unique opportunity to discover something you love. Don't be afraid to fail, every misstep is a valuable lesson that brings you closer to discovering your true passion. I never excelled at sports or music, but I discovered other passions that bring me joy.

Try New Activities:

- Make a list of activities you've always been curious about but haven't explored. These could include creative endeavors like pottery or photography, physical activities like hiking or yoga, or intellectual pursuits such as learning a new language. Several years ago, my husband and I took a leap of faith. After visiting Panama, we returned home, packed all our belongings, and moved to the Panamanian mountains with our two dogs, immersing ourselves in the Spanish language and culture.

What Makes You Happy:

- Reflect on experiences that bring you joy and energy. Notice the activities that make you lose track of time or ones you eagerly anticipate. These "flow" moments can strongly indicate your passion. If you're deeply engaged in writing, for instance, creative writing might be worth exploring.

Remember, finding your passion is a journey requiring patience and a willingness to explore.

EAT AND ENJOY – NOURISHING FOOD

Chicken is a versatile, protein-packed food essential to build and maintain muscle. Additionally, chicken is rich in essential amino acids, vitamins like B6 and B12, and minerals such as iron and zinc, which support overall health and vitality. Its lean nature also makes it ideal for those looking to manage their weight, without sacrificing flavor or satisfaction.

Experiment with Marinades and Rubs:

- Transform chicken flavor with different marinades and rubs. Simple marinades might include olive oil, lemon juice, garlic, and herbs, while dry rubs can feature spices like paprika, cumin, garlic powder, and oregano. Marinate for at least 30 minutes.

Try Different Cooking Methods:

- Change your cooking methods to discover different textures and flavors. Beyond grilling and baking, try roasting, sautéing, poaching, or slow cooking.

Incorporate International Flavors:

- Consider Italian, Indian, Thai, Mexican, and Mediterranean dishes. Chicken parmesan, chicken tikka masala, Thai chicken curry, Mexican chicken fajitas, or Greek souvlaki can turn your meals into a culinary adventure. Try the **Chicken Portobello Florentine.**

Make Use of Sauces and Toppings:

- Elevate chicken dishes with sauces and toppings like homemade salsa, guacamole, tzatziki, or chimichurri. Add variety with toppings such as avocado slices, nuts, and seeds.

Turn Leftovers into New Dishes:

- Repurpose leftover chicken into salads, wraps, soups, or pizzas. Shredded chicken is great for tacos, enchiladas, or even omelets.

With a variety of cooking techniques and flavors, you are less likely to become bored with plain, bland chicken.

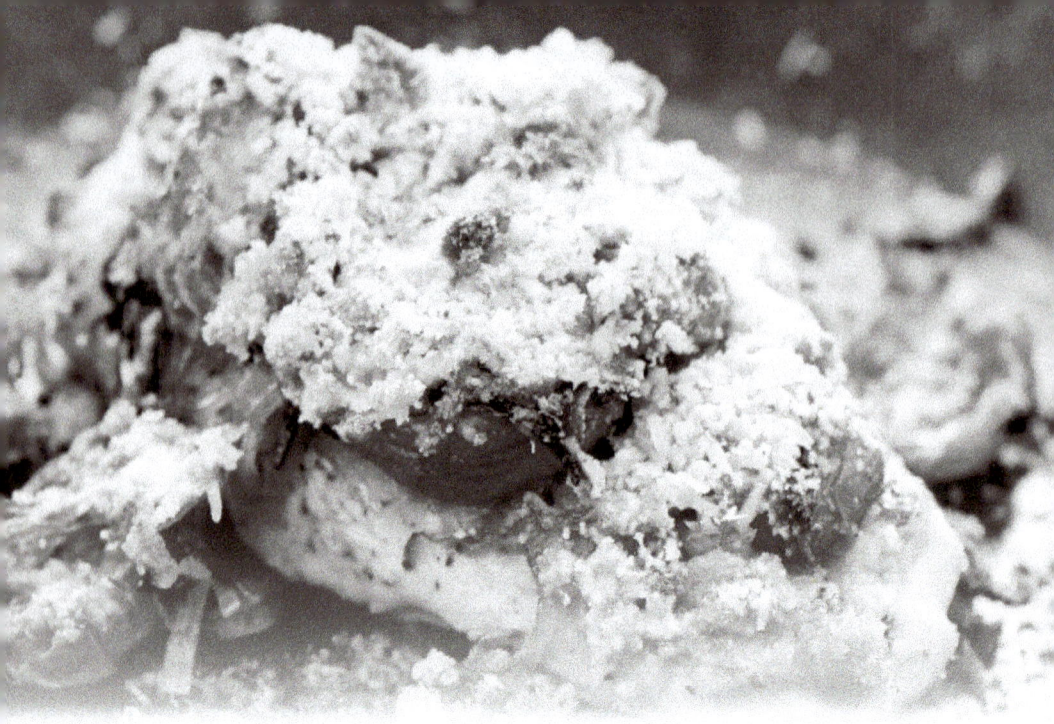

Chicken Portobello Florentine

4-6 servings

INGREDIENTS:

- ½ cup balsamic vinegar
- 3 Tablespoons olive oil + 2 Tablespoons for sautéing
- 1 Tablespoon honey
- 1 teaspoon Dijon mustard
- 1 teaspoon garlic powder
- 2 teaspoons Italian seasoning
- Salt and pepper
- 2 lb. boneless skinless chicken breasts, sliced into thin cutlets
- 8 oz. baby spinach
- 2 large portobello mushrooms, sliced thin
- 2 cups marinara sauce
- ½ cup shredded mozzarella cheese

PROCESS:

1. In a measuring cup, mix vinegar, olive oil, honey, Dijon, garlic, Italian seasoning, and salt and pepper to taste.

2. Put in a zip-top bag.

3. Reserve 3 T of marinade for mushrooms and pour the remaining marinade in the bag with the chicken. Massage chicken into marinade and put on a plate in the refrigerator for 30 minutes or up to 6 hours.

4. Put sliced mushrooms in a bowl and gently toss with reserved marinade.

5. Heat skillet with 2 T. olive oil until shimmery.

6. Add mushrooms and cook until soft. Remove from heat and drain.

7. Remove mushrooms from pan, add more oil if needed, and sauté spinach until wilted.

8. Remove chicken from marinade and cook and choose cooking method:

- Sauté: 3-5 minutes per side until no longer pink in the center.
- Bake: Preheat oven to 375°F. Put chicken in a baking dish and bake for 15-20 minutes until no longer pink in the center.
- Grill: Grill over medium heat 3-5 minutes per side until no longer pink in the center.

Top chicken breasts with sautéed spinach, sliced mushrooms, marinara sauce, and mozzarella cheese. Heat it in the oven or on the grill until cheese melts.

ACTIVITY – EMBRACE AND LOVE MOVEMENT

If you're interested in starting weight training but unsure where to begin, don't worry about buying expensive equipment or heading to the gym right away. You can start by using everyday household items like cans and jugs of water. A can of beans typically weighs around 1 lb., while a gallon of water weighs about 8 lbs.

Warm-Up:

- Always start with a warm-up to get your muscles ready for the workout. This could be a few minutes of walking, marching in place, or some light stretching.

Progress Gradually:

- Increase weight gradually as you become more comfortable and stronger. You can add more water to jugs or use larger cans. Focusing on correct form rather than lifting heavier weights helps prevent injury and ensure muscle groups are targeted.

Bicep Curls:

- Hold a can or jug in each hand, arms at your sides. Slowly bend your elbows, bringing the cans or jugs towards your shoulders. Lower and repeat.

Triceps Extensions:

- Hold a can or jug in both hands, arms overhead. Bend your elbows, lower the weight behind your head, straighten your arms and lift the weight back up.

Squats:

- Hold a can or jug in each hand, arms at your sides. Perform squats as you normally would, keeping your back straight and lowering down as if you are sitting into a chair. Ensure your knees do not go past your toes.

Consistency is key, aim to include these exercises 3-4 times a week.

KINDNESS – CULTIVATE IT IN YOUR DAILY LIFE

Begin cultivating kindness close to home. Embrace the well-known insurance company's slogan, *"Like a good neighbor, State Farm is there."* I grew up in the 1950s where neighbors helped each other. My mom always offered to watch the neighborhood kids, and we would hop rides to the local pool with our neighbors.

Offer to Mow Their Yard or Shovel Snow:

- Helping with yard work or snow removal is especially valuable to elderly neighbors or those with physical limitations.

Bring Over a Homemade Treat:

- Sharing homemade goodies can brighten someone's day. It's a thoughtful way to show that you care and provides an opportunity to connect and engage in conversation. Living in North Carolina's apple country, my neighbors Dave and Beth share apple homemade sauce every fall. My other neighbors Sharon and Anne, both great bakers, share cakes and cookies. We jokingly say they are trying to get us fat! Another neighbor, Kathy shares flower bulbs to help beautify the small neighborhood.

Help with Groceries:

- Offer to help your neighbors carry their groceries or heavy items into their home. This small act can be a great relief, particularly for those who struggle with mobility.

Share Surplus Produce:

- If you have a garden, share your surplus produce with your neighbors. Fresh fruits, vegetables, or herbs.

Take Time to Chat:

- The simplest act of kindness is taking the time to chat, A friendly conversation builds stronger relationships and creates a more supportive community.

In today's fast-paced world, these gestures foster a sense of belonging and connection.

Log Today's Activities and Experiences with The SPEAK Method

Use the questions or comments as a guide or write freely expressing your thoughts!

SELF-CARE – Did you schedule a honey/egg mask or maybe a professional facial?

_____
_____
_____
_____
_____
_____
_____
_____

PASSION – What new activities are you going to explore?

_____
_____
_____
_____
_____
_____
_____
_____

EAT AND ENJOY NOURISHING FOOD – Any new chicken recipes you plan on trying?

_____
_____
_____
_____
_____
_____
_____
_____
_____

ACTIVITY – What cans and jugs do you have set out so you can access them for weights?

_____
_____
_____
_____
_____
_____
_____
_____
_____

KINDNESS – Who are you choosing to be extra kind to, family, friends or neighbors?

_____
_____
_____
_____
_____
_____

ADDITIONAL NOTES

_____
_____
_____
_____
_____
_____

DAILY REPORT CARD OF LIFE – How did you SPEAK today?

Grade Your Day, no D's or F's Allowed!

- **A** – Amazing
- **B** – Better than yesterday
- **C** – Challenging but working on it

Interview
Anne Geyer - 85 Years Young

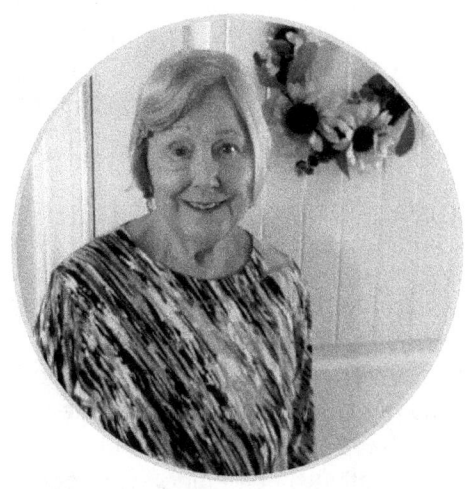

SELF-CARE – PRACTICE IT DAILY

Sleep is very important to me, so I make sure to get eight hours every night. I also pay close attention to my body; if I notice a problem, I try to figure it out on my own first. If I can't, I go to the doctor. To stay strong, I attend physical therapy, and the therapist always reminds me how young I am! Staying connected and social is a priority for me. When I moved here, I joined Welcome Wagon and became very active with my church. I love showing friends and family around the area when they visit.

PASSION – DISCOVER AND IGNITE IT

When my kids were in school, I worked part-time in food service at a college. When my husband retired and was home a lot, I jokingly said that I "didn't like it," so I went full-time! The best part of my job was working with the students. I continue my passion for helping young girls by volunteering with PEO Education, an organization dedicated to motivating, educating, and celebrating women. Through this organization, we assist young girls in finding colleges and provide career counseling. It keeps me young!

To learn more about PEO Education, go to peointernational.org

EAT AND ENJOY – NOURISHING FOOD

I mainly eat fresh fruits, vegetables, fish, and chicken, while limiting my red meat consumption. I love pickled items, including eggs, beets, and any kind of pickles. I often soak boiled eggs in the juice from pickled beets to make pretty, pink pickled eggs, which are said to be rich in probiotics. Additionally, I enjoy going out to eat with friends and family to explore local restaurants while making good choices and not overeating.

ACTIVITY – EMBRACE AND LOVE MOVEMENT

I am not one to sit around; I love to stay active. I used to bowl, but after being diagnosed with MS, I'm not as steady on my feet as I once was. Now, I spend my time working in my yard—planting, weeding, and watering the abundance of flowers around my house. I even save my zinnia seeds to plant next year. Many people comment that I have the most beautiful flowers in the neighborhood. I also stay active by cleaning and decorating my house for the holidays, both indoors and out. Additionally, I volunteer for socials at church and have enjoyed doing so for years.

KINDNESS – CULTIVATE IT IN YOUR DAILY LIFE

As an 85-year-old woman, I advise, "Kindness is the most important thing to have in your life. Why be ugly and mean when you can be kind?" I make it a point to talk to everyone I meet, believing there's always something good in every person. It's essential to make the best of life and always remember to be kind.

DAY 3

"Keep only those things that speak to your heart. Then take the plunge and discard all the rest."

Marie Kondo, Japanese organizing consultant and author

SELF-CARE – PRACTICE IT DAILY

A simple self-care practice is to start decluttering your space. This can have a profound impact on your mental clarity and stress levels. The process of decluttering is therapeutic, helping you let go of the past and make room for the new. My stepdaughter Brooke is a master of decluttering. She has organized my pantry numerous times, but I always seem to clutter it back up!

Start Small:

- Begin by tackling one area at a time, whether it's a room, a closet, or even a drawer. Sort items into categories: keep, donate, recycle, or discard. This sorting process helps in making clear decisions about what's truly necessary and valuable.

Emotional Attachments:

- Be mindful of the emotional attachment to items and ask yourself if each item serves a purpose or brings joy. This method, inspired by Marie Kondo's philosophy, helps in being intentional with what you keep in your living space. Letting go of items that no longer serve you can be freeing, providing a fresh start.

Organization Tips:

- Organize the items you keep in functional and efficient ways that make them easily accessible. Use storage solutions like bins, shelves, and drawer organizers to keep things tidy. Labeling storage can also help maintain order and make finding items easier.

Maintain Organization:

- Regularly maintaining a clutter-free space can enhance your focus and productivity. A clean, organized environment reduces distractions, making it easier to concentrate on tasks. This newfound efficiency can contribute to a more relaxed and enjoyable ambiance.

By clearing out unnecessary items, you're also creating a calmer, more focused decluttered mind.

PASSION – DISCOVER AND IGNITE IT

Recognizing your strengths is essential for uncovering your passion and purpose. Understanding what you excel at and enjoy enables you to align your activities with these strengths, resulting in greater satisfaction and success. This alignment creates a synergistic effect, fostering both personal and professional growth.

Identify Your Strengths:

- Start with an honest assessment of your abilities. Reflect on activities and tasks where you excel without significant effort. Consider the compliments and positive feedback you've received from others; external recognition can highlight strengths you might overlook.

Utilize Tests:

- Take a strengths assessment test, such as Gallup StrengthsFinder, for a structured analysis of your capabilities. These assessments provide valuable insights into your dominant talents.

Find Your Joy:

- Self-reflection is vital. Identify activities that give you a sense of achievement and fulfillment. For instance, if you find joy in organizing events, you likely have strong leadership and planning skills. If you lose track of time while painting or composing music, artistic talents could be among your strengths.

Leverage Strengths:

- Leverage strengths by seeking opportunities that allow you to use and develop them further. This could mean taking on new projects at work that align with your capabilities, volunteering in roles that utilize your talents, or starting personal projects that challenge and hone your skills.

Focusing on what you are naturally good at and enjoy will enhance your competence and bring greater joy and fulfillment

EAT AND ENJOY – NOURISHING FOOD

Listening to your body is a critical component of healthy eating. By paying attention to hunger and fullness cues, you can maintain a balanced diet. Recognizing these cues helps prevent both overeating and undereating.

Savor Your Food:

- Start by eating slowly and mindfully, allowing yourself to savor each bite. This enables you to detect when you feel satisfied rather than waiting until you feel overly full.

Why You are Hungry:

- Consider the difference between physical hunger and emotional hunger; the latter often leads to unhealthy eating habits. To differentiate, ask yourself if you're truly hungry or if you're eating out of boredom, stress, or other emotions.

Understanding Fullness:

- Your body gives fullness cues too. Aim to eat until you're about 80% full—this is typically when your body has had enough, but you haven't reached the point of discomfort. Remember, it takes about 20 minutes for your brain to register fullness.

Mindful Approach:

- By tuning into your body's signals, you're more likely to choose foods that meet its needs, rather than relying on external cues like the time or social situations.

Eat Good Fats:

- Good fat keeps you full longer. Incorporate avocados, olive oil, avocado oil and coconut oil into your meals. We had the pleasure of living amidst the avocado orchards near Fallbrook, California. Imagine getting ten avocados for just five dollars! We relished avocados in everything, including **Guacamole** and **Avocado Deviled Eggs.**

Our bodies speak to us, we just need to listen!

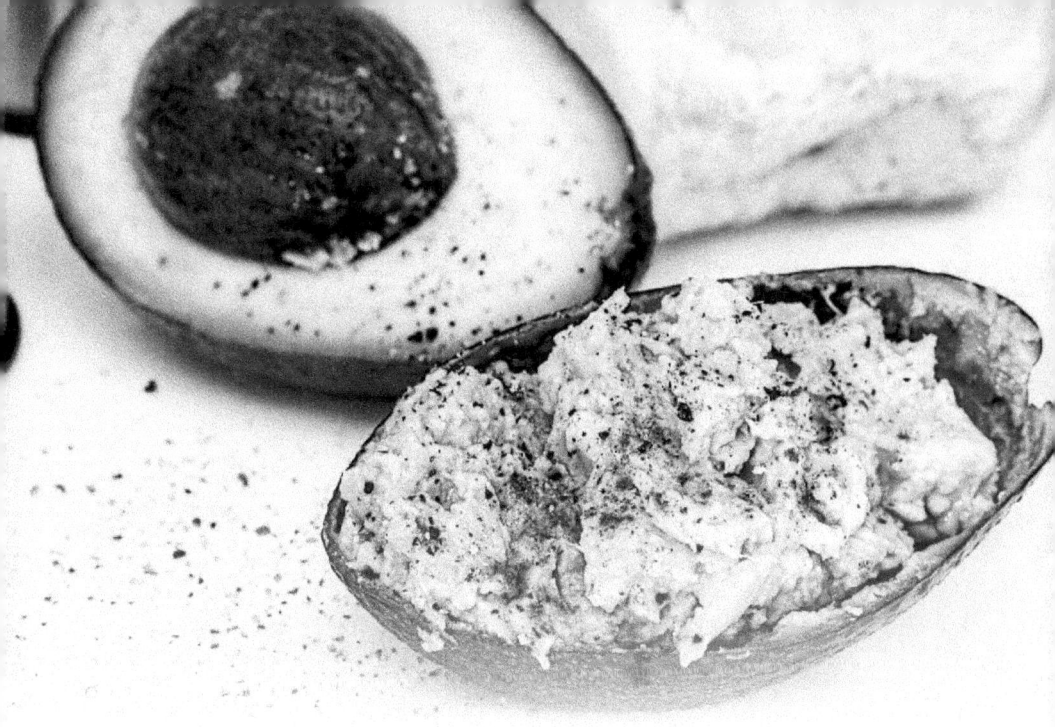

Guacamole

5-6 Servings

INGREDIENTS:

- 4 ripe avocados, peeled and mashed
- 1 teaspoon sea salt
- ½ teaspoon black pepper
- 1 lime, juiced
- 2 teaspoons garlic powder or two cloves, minced
- 3 Tablespoons fresh cilantro, diced
- 4 Roma tomatoes, diced
- ½ medium red onion, diced
- 1 small jalapeño pepper, diced (more or less for spice preference)

PROCESS:

1. Peel, seed, and mash avocado to a smooth consistency and add to a large bowl.
2. Dice onion, tomatoes, garlic, jalapeno pepper, and cilantro and add to the bowl.
3. Season with freshly squeezed lime juice and salt and pepper.

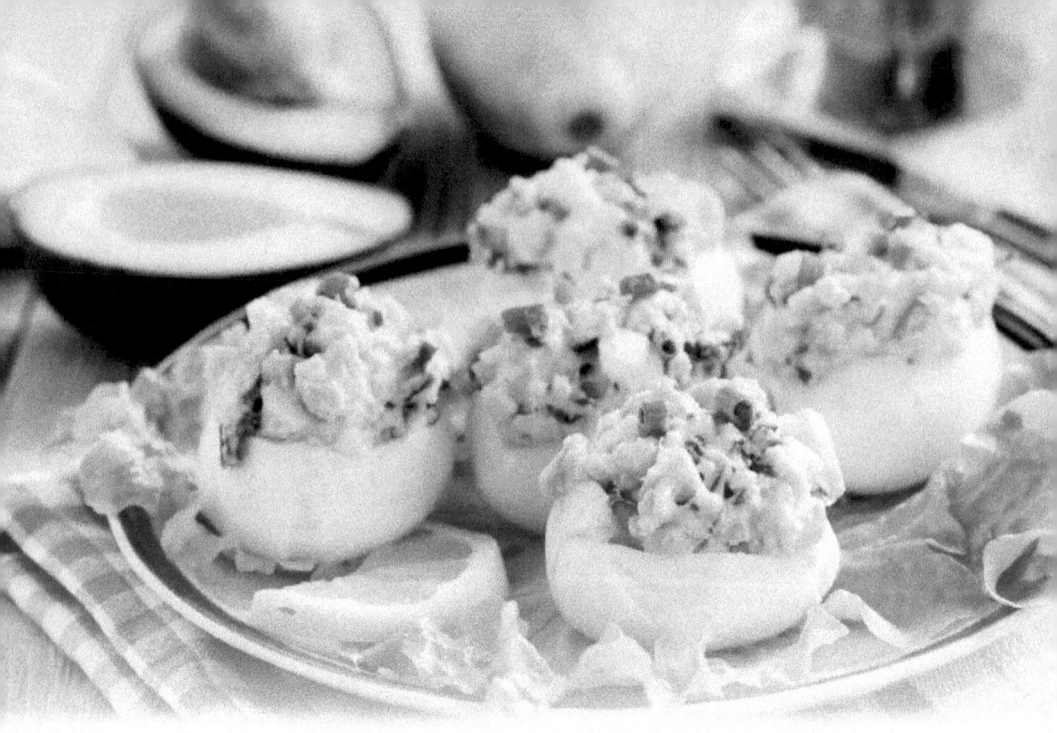

Avocado Deviled Eggs

4-6 Servings

INGREDIENTS:

- 6 hard-boiled eggs, peeled and halved
- 1 avocado - peeled, pitted, and diced
- 2 1/2 Tablespoons mayonnaise
- 2 teaspoons lime juice
- 1 clove garlic, crushed
- 1/8 teaspoon cayenne pepper (more or less for spice preference)
- Sea salt to taste
- 1 jalapeno pepper, sliced (optional)

PROCESS:

1. Scoop egg yolks into a bowl; add avocado, mayonnaise, lime juice, garlic, cayenne pepper, and salt. Mash egg yolk mixture until filling is evenly combined.
2. Spoon filling into a piping bag or plastic bag with a snipped corner. Pipe or scoop filling into each egg white; Top with optional jalapeno slice.

ACTIVITY – EMBRACE AND LOVE MOVEMENT

A simple activity is to incorporate stretching exercises throughout the day. Stretching is vital for maintaining flexibility, reducing muscle tension, and preventing injuries. Regular stretching helps to improve blood flow to the muscles, reduce stiffness, and enhance your range of motion. While writing this book, I made it a point to get up every hour for a stretch. I genuinely felt that my thinking improved after each session.

Begin Your Day:
- Start your day with a few gentle stretches to wake up your muscles and get your blood flowing. These can even be done in bed.

Take Breaks:
- Throughout the day, especially if you have a sedentary job, take short breaks to stretch different muscle groups. Focus on areas that tend to get tight from sitting, such as the neck, shoulders, back, and legs.

Keep it Simple:
- Simple stretches like reaching for your toes, doing neck rolls, and performing arm stretches can be very effective. Try standing up and sitting down, engaging your core.

Incorporate Stretching:
- Set reminders to stretch every hour or use prompts like standing and sitting during phone calls. Incorporating stretching into your daily routine can also reduce stress and improve posture. Remember to hold each stretch for 15-30 seconds and avoid bouncing to prevent injury.

Remember to Breathe:
- Deep breathing during stretching can enhance its benefits by helping to further relax the body and the brain.

Incorporating stretching into your daily routine enhances your overall physical well-being, maintains your body's flexibility and strength, and promotes mental acuity.

KINDNESS – CULTIVATE IT IN YOUR DAILY LIFE

A simple act of kindness is to compliment customer service representatives. We are usually quick to recognize the bad but rarely acknowledge the good. Having worked in the customer service industry for over 30 years, I deeply appreciate good service and consistently strive to practice it.

Express Appreciation:

- When you receive excellent service, take a moment to express your appreciation sincerely. These professionals often deal with challenging situations and long hours. A kind word can make a significant difference in their day.

Be Specific:

- Giving detailed compliments is particularly meaningful. For instance, you might say, "Thank you for your patience and help today; it made a big difference," or "You handled that situation with such professionalism." Offering detailed feedback, highlights what they did well and shows that you genuinely noticed their efforts.

Give Manager Feedback:

- Ask to speak to a manager, and with a smile, say, "I know customers usually ask to speak to you when service is bad. I want to let you know what great service your staff gave today!"

Online Reviews:

- When possible, leave positive feedback through company surveys or online review platforms to ensure their supervisors recognize their hard work.

Compliment in Public:

- Too many times we hear customers loudly complaining in public. In contrast, publicly complimenting great service in front of other colleagues and customers can be very empowering to the server.

Consistently expressing gratitude for customer service fosters a culture of appreciation and respect.

Log Today's Activities and Experiences with The SPEAK Method

Use the questions or comments as a guide or write freely expressing your thoughts!

SELF-CARE – What areas are you going to declutter first?

_____
_____
_____
_____
_____
_____
_____

PASSION – List some of your best strengths.

_____
_____
_____
_____
_____
_____
_____
_____

EAT AND ENJOY NOURISHING FOOD – In listening to your body while eating, what did you discover? Are you eating too much or wrong food for emotional reasons?

___

ACTIVITY – What are of your body are you going to stretch first?

___

KINDNESS – What were your customer service interactions on the phone, in a chat or in person. How were you kind?

_____
_____
_____
_____
_____
_____

ADDITIONAL NOTES

_____
_____
_____
_____
_____
_____

DAILY REPORT CARD OF LIFE – How did you SPEAK today?

Grade Your Day, no D's or F's Allowed!

- **A** – Amazing
- **B** – Better than yesterday
- **C** – Challenging but working on it

DAY 4

"Anyone who stops learning is old, whether at twenty or eighty. Anyone who keeps learning stays young."
- Henry Ford

SELF-CARE – PRACTICE IT DAILY

Laughter is one of the most invaluable tools for self-care that you can easily and enjoyably integrate into your day. "Laughter is the best medicine," providing numerous benefits for both physical and mental health. Laughter triggers the release of endorphins, the body's natural feel-good chemicals and helps reduce the stress hormone cortisol, boost immune function, and improve cardiovascular health.

Be Around Fun People:

- Spend time with friends and family who have a good sense of humor; their laughter can be contagious, lightening your mood and creating lasting, joyful memories. My favorite brother-in-law, Mike, had the most infectious laugh. Though he has sadly passed, his laughter lives on through his family. Remember to share joyous moments and laughter with your children.

Things that Make You Laugh:

- Engage in activities that naturally induce laughter, such as playing games, or reminiscing about funny experiences. Watch a funny movie, you're giving your body and mind a valuable boost.

Tell Jokes or Funny Stories:

- Make a point to share funny stories and jokes. It simultaneously enhances brain function, as you need to remember the punchlines! No matter how silly, funny stories or jokes make us laugh. I recently spent time with my 4 ½- year-old great niece who loves "knock, knock" jokes. Some of them did not make sense but all of them got her and I laughing profusely!

Incorporating laughter into your daily routine, or simply smiling at the little absurdities in life doesn't just benefit your health, it also strengthens social bonds.

PASSION – DISCOVER AND IGNITE IT

Taking classes, whether online or at a local community college, is an excellent way to identify your passions. These educational opportunities allow you to explore a diverse range of subjects in a structured, low-pressure environment. My background was science and food service, I never liked to write. When I decided to share my passion for health and healthy food, I did some online writing classes. I then took a couple of courses at the local community college where I learned valuable lessons from not only the instructors but also my fellow students.

Personal Development Courses:

- These courses often include topics like goal setting, self-awareness, and discovering your strengths. They are designed to help you understand yourself better and identify what truly excites you.

Entrepreneurship and Business Classes:

- If you're interested in creating something of your own, these classes can help you learn how to start and manage a business. They also often include exercises to identify your core passions and values.

Skills-Based Courses:

- Whether it's writing, painting, cooking, music or carpentry, trying out different courses can help you discover new interests and areas you're passionate about.

Mindfulness and Meditation Classes:

- These classes can help you connect with your true self by fostering a deeper sense of inner peace and awareness, often making it easier to see what ignites your passion.

Ultimately, taking classes is not just about gaining knowledge but also about sparking curiosity and finding what truly excites you.

EAT AND ENJOY – NOURISHING FOOD

Expand your culinary experience with Mother Nature's original medicine - herbs and spices. They offer vibrant flavors and a wealth of antioxidants, vitamins, and minerals. Replacing excess salt and processed sugar with herbs and spices adds flavor and nutrition.

I had the chance to stay on an organic ginger and turmeric farm in Costa Rica's rainforest. During a forest walk, a local guide shared the medicinal plants his family has used for generations, revealing remedies for headaches, digestion issues, pain relief, and more.

Brain Fog:

- Rosemary has been shown to support memory and concentration. Experiencing afternoon brain fog, sniff your rosemary plant or put in your marinades!

Natural Blood Sugar Support:

- Cinnamon supports healthy blood sugar levels, making it a great addition for those watching their sugar intake. Add to your morning coffee, tea, or oatmeal.

Support Digestion:

- Cumin, ginger and cayenne support a healthy digestive system and may boost your metabolism, aiding in weight loss.

Anti-Inflammatory:

- Ginger contains gingerol to support digestion and reduce inflammation. Put ginger in a tea or in a stir-fry with **Orange Honey Teriyaki Sauce.** Turmeric, rich in curcumin, has also been shown to combat chronic inflammation. Make a golden milk tea with turmeric.

Fresh vs. Dried:

- Whenever possible, opt for fresh herbs, add fresh basil, parsley, or cilantro to your salads. When using dried herbs sauté or infuse them in olive oil to bring out both the flavor and health benefits.

Experiment with different combinations and try making your own unique spice blend.

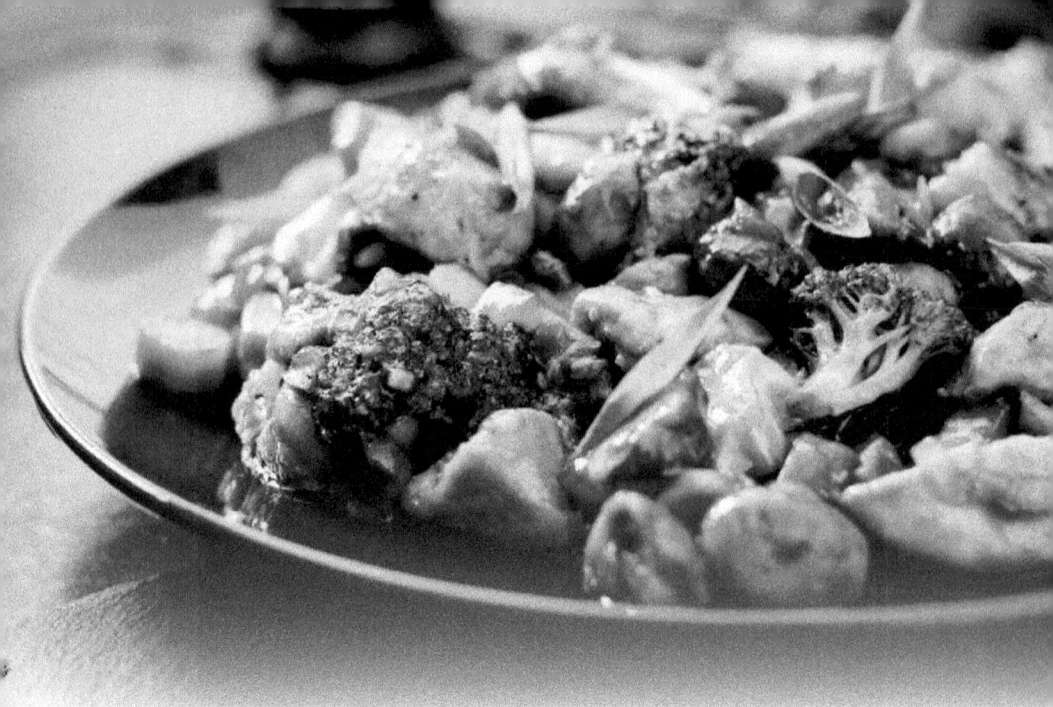

Orange Honey Teriyaki Sauce

INGREDIENTS:

- 2/3 cup tamari or soy sauce
- 1/4 cup rice vinegar
- 1 orange, juiced and zested
- 1/2 cup water
- 2/3 cup honey
- 1/4 teaspoon ground ginger
- 1/4 teaspoon garlic powder
- 3 Tablespoons arrowroot or cornstarch mixed with 2 Tablespoons water

PROCESS:

1. Heat all ingredients except for the arrowroot or cornstarch mixture and water mixture in small saucepan until it just begins to boil.
2. Mix arrowroot with water and slowly add to pan while whisking continually. Do not allow it to boil after mixture is added. If sauce is too thick you may thin with water or chicken stock. Serve over stir fry or toss into stir fry. Store in the fridge for up to 2 weeks.

Serving Suggestions:

- Drizzle on steamed vegetables.
- Stir-fry meat or seafood of choice with vegetables. Add teriyaki sauce and serve over rice.
- Add 2 Tablespoons olive or avocado oil per 2 Tablespoons teriyaki sauce and use as an Asian salad dressing.

ACTIVITY – EMBRACE AND LOVE MOVEMENT

Taking a short walk after meals is an easy and effective method to increase your daily physical activity and support a healthy weight. Walking post-meals boosts the production of serotonin and endorphins, which enhance mood and alleviate stress.

Did you ever want to take a nap after Thanksgiving dinner? I sure did! To combat that post-meal drowsiness, our family now takes a refreshing walk after Thanksgiving meal. This new tradition not only helps us feel more energized but also provides a wonderful opportunity to bond and enjoy the crisp autumn air.

Aid Digestion:

- Walking after eating helps stimulate digestion, prevents bloating, and aids in controlling blood sugar levels. Start with a 10–15-minute walk at a moderate pace and build up the time and pace over time.

Your Route:

- Choose a pleasant route, such as around your neighborhood, a nearby park, or in bad weather, even up and down the corridors of your home or workplace.

Clear the Mind:

- Walking after meals helps you decompress and clear your mind, making it a great time for reflection or conversation with a walking partner.

Consistent Schedule:

- To make it a habit, schedule your walks immediately after meals, turning them into a consistent part of your daily routine.

Small changes, like incorporating a post-meal walk, can make a big difference in your overall health and quality of life. Walk more and stress less!

KINDNESS – CULTIVATE IT IN YOUR DAILY LIFE

"Paying it forward" involves performing a kind act for someone else in response to a kind act you received, creating a ripple effect of kindness. This simple yet powerful concept spreads positivity beyond the initial gesture.

Start Small:

- Pay for the coffee of the person behind you in line, help a mom with kids carry out her groceries, talk to a lonely-looking elderly person, give a friend a ride.

Encourage Others:

- When someone thanks you, remind them to pay it forward by doing something kind for the next person.

Share your Pay-it-Forward Stories:

Sharing your stories will inspire others to pay it forward.

One of my personal simple Pay-it-Forward stories: One Sunday morning at the local coffee shop, I noticed two soldiers sitting with serious expressions. I went to the counter and purchased a small gift card. When I approached them, I asked where they were from. They shared that they were from nearby but were about to be deployed to different locations and didn't know when they'd see each other again. I offered them the gift card as a thank-you for their service, hoping they could enjoy one more cup of coffee together before parting. They expressed their gratitude and mentioned that no one had ever done such a kind act for them before. I simply asked them to pay it forward. They smiled and promised they would.

These small gestures remind us of our shared humanity. Keep the kindness chain going!

Log Today's Activities and Experiences with The SPEAK Method

Use the questions or comments as a guide or write freely expressing your thoughts!

SELF-CARE – Who and what made you laugh today?

_____
_____
_____
_____
_____
_____
_____
_____

PASSION – What classes are you going to explore?

_____
_____
_____
_____
_____
_____
_____
_____

EAT AND ENJOY NOURISHING FOOD – List some new spices you want to try.

_____
_____
_____
_____
_____
_____
_____
_____
_____

ACTIVITY – Where did you walk after one of your meals. How did you feel?

_____
_____
_____
_____
_____
_____
_____
_____
_____

KINDNESS – List ways you plan on Paying it Forward and with whom.

_____
_____
_____
_____
_____
_____

ADDITIONAL NOTES

_____
_____
_____
_____
_____
_____

DAILY REPORT CARD OF LIFE – How did you SPEAK today?

Grade Your Day, no D's or F's Allowed!

- **A** – Amazing
- **B** – Better than yesterday
- **C** – Challenging but working on it

DAY 5

"Have the courage to follow your heart and intuition. They somehow already know what you truly want to become."
Steve Jobs

SELF-CARE – PRACTICE IT DAILY

Spending time with pets is a wonderful self-care tip and can be incredibly therapeutic. Animals provide unconditional love and companionship, which can significantly reduce stress and alleviate feelings of loneliness. Our Westie, Mollie Mae, brings us joy daily with her silly antics, like watching TV. It's no surprise that her favorite movie is "A Dog's Purpose."

Benefits of Pets:

- Engaging with pets, whether through play, petting, walking or simply sitting with them, has been shown to lower blood pressure and stimulate the release of serotonin and oxytocin, chemicals that naturally enhance mood and create a sense of well-being.

Find a Pet:

- If you don't own a pet, don't worry! There are numerous ways to benefit from animal interaction. Visiting friends who have pets, volunteering at an animal shelter, or participating in animal-assisted therapy programs are excellent alternatives. Offer to walk a neighbor's dog or better yet, offer to pet sit if they are going away for the weekend.

  When I lived in the mountains of Panama, I volunteered at a spay and neuter clinic called Amigos de Animales. Assisting with the stray dog situation and helping residents with affordable care was incredibly rewarding. I gained more from the experience than the dogs I cared for during recovery.

Activity and Routines:

- Walking a dog or grooming a pet also provides physical exercise and a sense of routine, both of which are beneficial for mental and physical health.

To have a happier and more balanced life,
spend time with animals.

PASSION – DISCOVER AND IGNITE IT

There is truly something to be said about "trusting your gut." Harnessing your intuition to uncover your true passion involves tuning into your inner voice and trusting your gut feelings and often guides us towards what truly excites and fulfills us.

Quiet Time:

- Start by creating quiet time for yourself. Practices such as meditation, journaling, or walking in nature can help calm your mind and open yourself up to intuitive insights. Pay attention to recurring thoughts and feelings.

Daydreaming:

- What activities spark joy? What subjects do you find yourself daydreaming about? These are often clues to what your passions might be.

Trust First Instincts:

- Listen to your body's reactions. When you think about different activities or career paths, notice how your body responds. A sense of excitement or a surge of energy can be a strong indicator that something resonates with your core desires. Don't overthink. Trust your first reactions.

Connect the Dots:

- Reflect on past experiences where you felt in the flow, fully engaged, and content. What were you doing in those moments? Our intuition often connects these seemingly unrelated events to form a clear picture of our true interests.

Outside Perspective:

- Seek feedback from trusted friends, family, or mentors who know you well. Sometimes, hearing an outside perspective can help validate what your intuition is telling you.

Remember, finding your passion is a journey, not a destination. Trusting your intuition can lead to small steps that gradually guide you closer to your true calling.

EAT AND ENJOY – NOURISHING FOOD

Planning meals and prepping protein are powerful strategies that can significantly enhance your commitment to healthy eating and save money.

Balanced Nutrition:

- Meal planning helps ensure balanced nutrient intake and portion control, crucial for managing weight and overall health.
- Protein is vital for muscle repair, immune function, and energy levels. Having protein readily available supports balanced meals and snacks, aiding in the inclusion of the good complex carbs - vegetables, whole grains, and healthy fats.
- Meal planning and protein prepping can save time, reduce stress, streamline grocery shopping, decrease food waste, and provide more time for other important activities.
- Homemade meals often contain less added sugar, sodium, and unhealthy fats compared to processed foods.

Ways to Prep Proteins:

- Grill extra chicken, portion it into snack-size baggies, and refrigerate for 2-3 days or freeze.
- Perfect for stir-fry, salad, or soup.
- Cook ground turkey, chicken, or lean beef. Season half with taco seasoning and half with Italian seasoning. Portion for quick tacos or spaghetti.
- Make beans or lentils for meal bowls, burritos, or soups.
- Prepare and freeze **Cheesy Zucchini and Red Pepper Egg Bites** for a quick breakfast.

Keep Protein Snacks on Hand:

- Pre-portion nuts and seeds to avoid overeating.
- Keep Greek yogurt and cottage cheese available.
- Boil eggs for snacks, egg salad, or to top salads.
- Make your own "Snackable's" with meat, cheese, and whole-grain crackers.

Start with simple meal planning then try more adventurous choices over time.

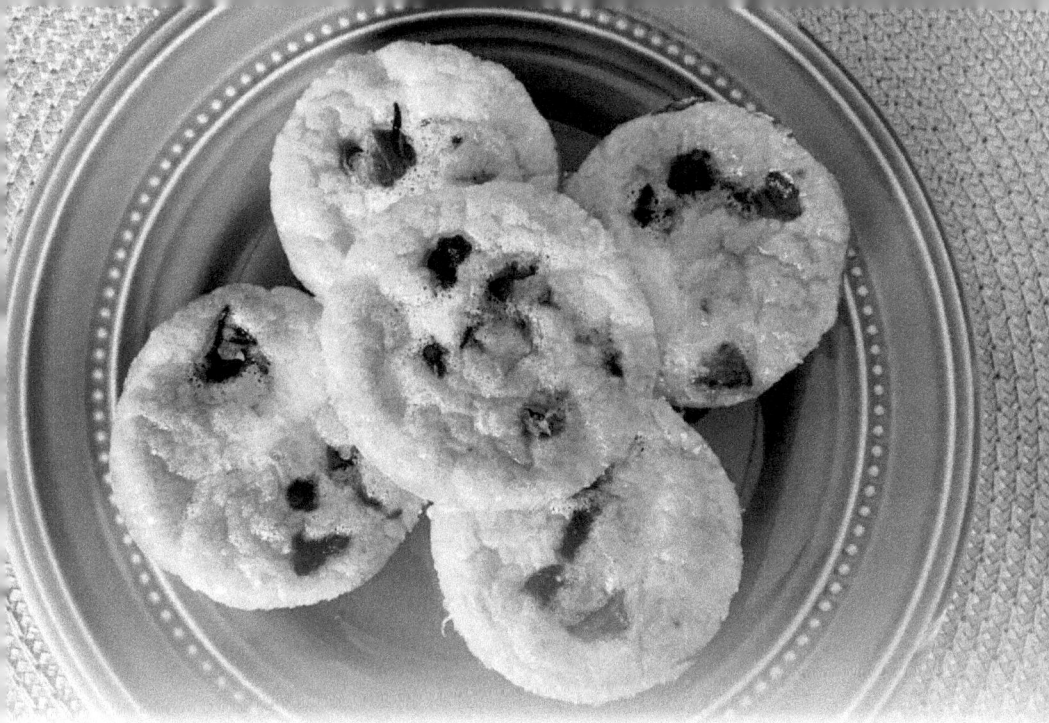

Cheesy Zucchini and Red Pepper Egg Bites

Makes 12 bites

INGREDIENTS:

- 8 eggs
- 2 cups shredded Swiss cheese
- 1 1/2 cups cottage cheese
- 1 cup crumbled feta cheese
- 3 cups spiralized or shredded zucchini
- 1 red pepper diced
- Salt & pepper, to taste
- Oil or cooking spray to coat muffin tins
- 3-4 Tablespoons fresh basil, rough chopped

PROCESS:

1. Pre-heat oven to 350°F
2. Spiralized or shredded zucchini

3. Beat eggs in medium bowl. Add shredded cheese, cottage cheese, ½ the feta, salt, and pepper.
4. Spray a muffin tin with olive oil spray and set on a sheet pan
5. Divide the zucchini equally in the muffin tins.
6. Fill the tins almost to the top with the egg mixture.
7. Top diced red peppers and remaining feta.
8. Bake in oven for 30 minutes, or until the center of the egg bites are just set.
9. Remove from oven and add fresh basil. Let cool for 5 minutes, then use a spatula or fork to carefully remove them from the muffin tin.
10. Store the egg bites in the fridge for several days.
11. Reheat in the microwave or warm in the oven.
12. Also freezes well. Put in single layer in zip loc baggie.

ACTIVITY – EMBRACE AND LOVE MOVEMENT

Did you ever hula hoop as a kid? I did, and we used to have contests to see who could keep it going the longest! This energetic exercise engages your core, bolsters coordination, and enhances cardiovascular health. I was 7 years old when the hula hoops came out and begged my parents to get one!

How to Pick a Hula Hoop:

- Select a hula hoop that suits your height and skill level. The ideal hoop should reach between your waist and chest when stood vertically. Pick out your favorite color. If you don't like red and you have a red hula hoop, you are less likely to use it!

Start Simple:

- Begin with the basics of waist hooping: stand with your feet shoulder-width apart and gently rock your hips back and forth, maintaining a rhythmic motion to keep the hoop spinning.

New Tricks:

- As you gain confidence and proficiency, you can experiment with new tricks and moves, challenging yourself and adding variety to your routine.

How Long to Hula Hoop:

- An initial goal of hula hooping for 10-15 minutes a day is a great starting point, gradually extending the duration as you become more comfortable and skilled.

Multi-tasking:

- Incorporating upbeat music can amplify the enjoyment, turning your hooping session into a lively dance-like activity. Or put on your favorite recorded movie or listen to a book, time will fly by!

Hula hooping offers an excellent way to lighten your mood and inject some playfulness into your routine.

KINDNESS – CULTIVATE IT IN YOUR DAILY LIFE

Two of the most powerful words in any language are thank you. Whether you say, "Thank You," "Gracias," "Merci," "Grazie," "Danke," "khob khun" in Thailand, or express thanks in any other language, this simple yet powerful act of kindness with gratitude can have a significant positive impact. Making it a habit to thank people genuinely and frequently acknowledges their efforts and contributions, which can uplift their mood and strengthen your relationships.

Words of Appreciation:

- Whether you thank a colleague for their hard work, a friend for their support, or a stranger for a small act of kindness, your words of appreciation can make a lasting impression.

Personalize It:

- Personalizing thank-you messages adds extra warmth and sincerity. Instead of a generic thank you, specify what you are grateful for, such as, "Thank you for staying late to help me with the project," or "Thanks for opening the door for me- I was not sure how I was going to do it with my hands full." This specificity shows that you are truly attentive and appreciative of their actions.

Writing it Down:

- For an even deeper impact, consider writing a thank-you note or email. This additional effort can demonstrate that you genuinely value their help.

Public Thank You:

- Acknowledging someone's contributions publicly, whether in a team meeting or a social media post, can amplify their sense of appreciation and further boost morale.

Saying thank you not only benefits the recipient but also cultivates a positive mindset within you. Say thank you more and the world will be a happier place.

Log Today's Activities and Experiences with The SPEAK Method

Use the questions or comments as a guide or write freely expressing your thoughts!

SELF-CARE – How did you spend time with a pet? If you don't own a pet, list neighbors' pets and a time to offer to walk them.

_____
_____
_____
_____
_____
_____
_____
_____

PASSION – What is "your gut" telling you to pursue?

_____
_____
_____
_____
_____
_____
_____
_____

EAT AND ENJOY NOURISHING FOOD – What meals are you planning for the week?

_____
_____
_____
_____
_____
_____
_____
_____

ACTIVITY – Got your hula hoop? Before you get it practice air hooping – pretend you have one and it will get you ready for the real thing.

_____
_____
_____
_____
_____
_____
_____
_____

KINDNESS – Who did you thank today?

_____
_____
_____
_____
_____
_____

ADDITIONAL NOTES

_____
_____
_____
_____
_____
_____

DAILY REPORT CARD OF LIFE – How did you SPEAK today?

Grade Your Day, no D's or F's Allowed!

    A – Amazing
    B – Better than yesterday
    C – Challenging but working on it

DAY 6

"You aren't wealthy until you have something money can't buy."
Garth Brooks

SELF-CARE – PRACTICE IT DAILY

A simple self-care ritual involves basking in natural sunlight, which is essential for both your physical and mental well-being. Whether you're at the beach or in your backyard, getting outdoors is a vital component of maintaining good health.

Elevates Vitamin D Levels:

- Helps maintain strong bones, a robust immune system, and a stable mood.

Daily Outdoor Time:

- Aim for 15-30 minutes outdoors each day, preferably in the morning or late afternoon when the sun's rays are gentler.

Activities:

- Engage in walking, gardening, or simply relaxing in the sun. If outdoors for an extended period, protect your skin with sunscreen or wear long sleeves and a hat. Gardening has become my favorite form of self-care. Each morning, I spend time in my garden, feeling the soil and nurturing my plants. This simple act brings me peace, teaches patience, and connects me with nature

Regulates Circadian Rhythm:

- Circadian rhythm is our body's natural 24-hour cycle that regulates sleep, wakefulness, and other physiological processes. This internal clock responds to external cues like light and darkness, helping to ensure that we sleep well at night and stay alert during the day.

Indoor Alternative:

- On days when you can't get outdoors, sitting by a sunny window can also be beneficial.

Mental Well-Being:

- Natural light exposure can significantly boost your mood, increase energy levels, and sharpen mental clarity.

Embrace the outdoors and let natural sunlight work its magic on your body and mind.

PASSION – DISCOVER AND IGNITE IT

Transforming thoughts into actions to identify your passion starts with writing things down. Consistent journaling can help piece together the puzzle of your true passions and lead you to a more fulfilling and purpose-driven life.

Years ago, I traveled with a doctor who emphasized the importance of taking notes during his seminars on natural health. He would often say, "This is a writer downer". There is power in the written word.

Get a Journal:
- Choose one in your favorite color and size.

Daily or Weekly Journaling:
- Set a specific time to write freely without judgment. Reflect on your daily activities, noting what made you feel most alive and engaged. Ask, "What did I enjoy doing today?" or "What made me feel excited or fulfilled?"

Write About Dreams and Aspirations:
- Describe in detail the life you envision for yourself, including activities and people.

Create Lists:
- List activities, subjects, or experiences that have always intrigued you or that you've wanted to try, recognizing recurring themes.

Self-Reflection:
- Write about your achievements and consider which ones you enjoyed working towards the most. Reflect on strengths and skills you love using.

Capture Spontaneous Ideas:
- Use your journal to note any spontaneous ideas or inspirations throughout the day.

    Hint: Create a note section on your phone to 'talk to text' for spontaneous ideas. At the end of each day, write them down in your journal.

By recording your thoughts, experiences, and observations, you can generate insights that will spark your passion.

EAT AND ENJOY – NOURISHING FOOD

Growing up, did you enjoy the classic comfort food, macaroni salad made with white pasta and a generous helping of mayonnaise? While undeniably delicious, traditional macaroni salad often lacks the nutritional benefits that we strive for in our meals today. As we become more health-conscious, it's time to give this beloved dish a nutritious makeover.

Healthy Pasta Alternatives:

- Whole wheat pasta has more nutrients and pairs well with robust sauces.
- Gluten-free or lentil pastas are incredibly tasty, and chickpea provides over 20 grams of protein per serving while tasting remarkably like white pasta. I have even fooled my pasta loving husband with chickpea pasta. Look for an upcoming Chicken Parmesan recipe with chickpea pasta.

Enhance Salads:

- Incorporate plenty of vegetables and toss with a simple herb vinaigrette. Red peppers add vitamin C, and garlic boosts immune and cardiovascular health. Using olive oil in the dressing supports a healthy cardiovascular system. Try the **Mediterranean Pasta Salad**, packed with fresh vegetables, a healthy pasta, and a light, flavorful dressing.

Additional Alternatives:

- Zucchini noodles ("zoodles") are low-carb and nutrient-rich. Get a small low-cost spiralizer online and make sweet potato or winter squash noodles.

Preparation Tip:

- Cook pasta in salted water, stir frequently, rinse with cold water, and toss with olive oil. This cooking method keeps the pasta from sticking and allows refrigerator storage for 2-3 days.

Consider healthier pasta, sauce and dressing as alternatives to make your favorite dishes both delicious and nourishing.

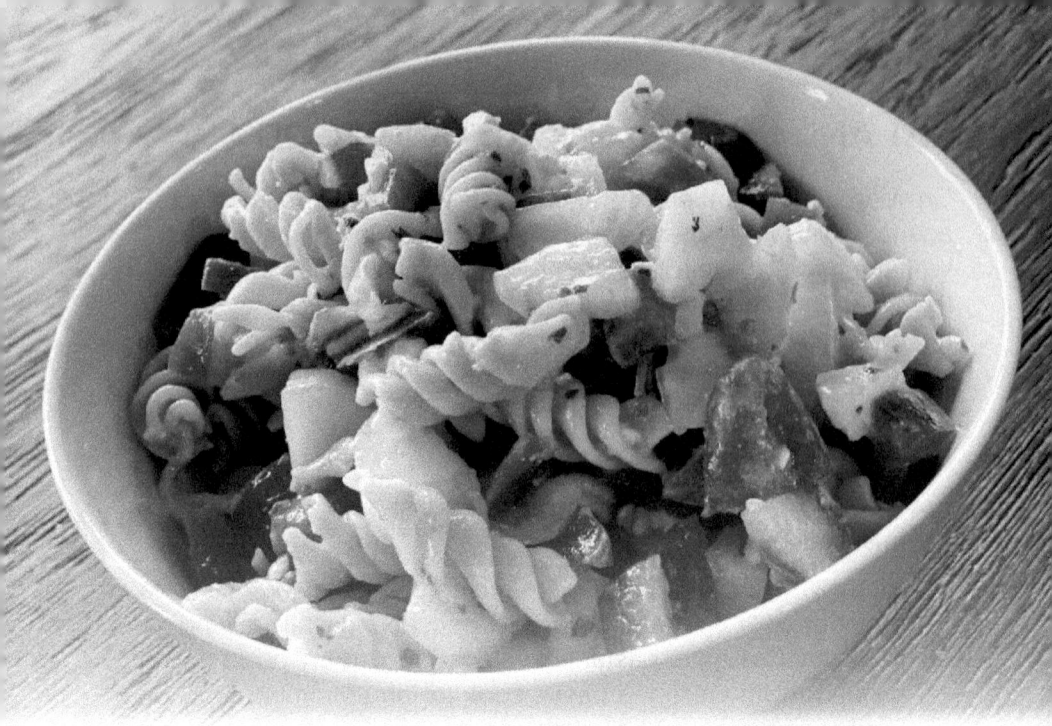

Mediterranean Pasta Salad

6-8 Servings

INGREDIENTS:

- 2 large cucumbers, diced
- 12-15 grape tomatoes, diced
- 2 large bell peppers, diced
- 8 oz. pasta (whole wheat or gluten-free: shells, spirals, or penne)
- 4 oz. crumbled Feta cheese
- 1/4 cup extra virgin olive oil
- Juice of 2 lemons
- 1 teaspoon sea salt
- 1 Tablespoon dried parsley or 3 tbsp chopped fresh parsley
- 1 teaspoon dried basil or 1 tbsp fresh chopped basil
- 1 teaspoon dried oregano or 1 tbsp chopped fresh oregano
- Sea salt and ground pepper to taste

PROCESS:

1. Prepare pasta according to package directions. Rinse well with cold water and drain.
2. Combine olive oil, lemon juice, and spices in a large bowl.
3. Add chopped vegetables, pasta, and feta. Stir well to combine.

HINT: Chickpea or red lentil pasta add extra protein, making this dish a complete meal.

ACTIVITY – EMBRACE AND LOVE MOVEMENT

Pacing around is a simple physical activity with numerous benefits. It can help clear your mind, boost creativity, and improve focus. Additionally, it offers a convenient way to break up periods of inactivity, keeping you energized throughout the day. As an accessible form of movement, pacing requires no special equipment or preparation, allowing you to engage in physical activity anytime and anywhere.

Boost Mental Clarity:
- Enhances blood flow to the brain, improving cognitive function and the flow of ideas.

Stimulate Creativity:
- Shakes up thinking patterns, breaks mental blocks and makes brainstorming more dynamic. **Disclosure:** I have paced around many hours while writing this book!

Increase Physical Activity:
- Incorporate light movement by pacing in a safe, open space such as a hallway, room, or office.

Voice Thoughts Aloud:
- While pacing, articulate ideas out loud to clarify thinking and reveal new insights.

Take Notes or Record Ideas:
- Keep a notebook handy or use your phone to jot down or record ideas while pacing.

Combine with Stretching:
- Integrate stretching into pacing for additional benefits.

Develop a Productive Habit:
- Encourages an active, innovative approach to problem-solving and supports better mental health.

Making pacing a habit during brainstorming fosters a more creative and effective approach to complex tasks while keeping you active. Combining movement with thought maximizes problem-solving potential and keeps your body engaged.

KINDNESS – CULTIVATE IT IN YOUR DAILY LIFE

Patience is a profound act of kindness that can significantly impact our relationships and personal well-being. Daily, practicing patience means giving others the time and space they need without rushing or pressuring them.

Supportive Work Environment:

- Allow a struggling coworker ample time to explain their point during meetings. This demonstrates understanding and respect, creating a supportive work environment.

Empathetic Relationships:

- In personal relationships, patience manifests when we listen to loved ones without interrupting, waiting for them to articulate their feelings and thoughts. This act validates their experiences and fosters stronger, more empathetic connections.

Nurturing Family Atmosphere:

- For parents or grandparents, patience with children as they learn, and grow is fundamental. Offering gentle guidance and understanding during moments of frustration can boost a child's confidence.

Customer Service Virtue:

- Most of us have worked in customer service where patience can truly be a virtue. Customer service interactions highlight how meaningful patience can be. When they remain calm and composed while addressing a frustrated client's concerns, it often diffuses the situation and leads to a more positive resolution.

Public Patience:

- In public spaces, patience can be shown by waiting calmly in long lines or aiding with elderly or disabled individuals without showing signs of impatience or frustration.

Ultimately, patience as an act of kindness not only benefits others but also enriches our own lives by reducing stress, building empathy, and fostering a more compassionate society.

Record Today's Activities and Experiences with The SPEAK Method

Use the questions or comments as a guide or write freely expressing your thoughts!

SELF-CARE – How long did you get outside today and did you feel refreshed?

_____
_____
_____
_____
_____
_____

PASSION – Did you purchase a journal? Until it arrives, take notes to transfer to your beautiful journal.

_____
_____
_____
_____
_____
_____
_____

EAT AND ENJOY NOURISHING FOOD – How do you plan to remake a pasta recipe?

_____
_____
_____
_____
_____
_____
_____
_____
_____

ACTIVITY – Did you consciously pace around today? What activities did you do while pacing?

_____
_____
_____
_____
_____
_____
_____
_____

KINDNESS – What tested your patience today and how did you handle the situation?

ADDITIONAL NOTES

DAILY REPORT CARD OF LIFE – How did you SPEAK today?

Grade Your Day, no D's or F's Allowed!

- **A** – Amazing
- **B** – Better than yesterday
- **C** – Challenging but working on it

DAY 7

> "Healthy boundaries are not walls. They are the gates and fences that allow you to enjoy the beauty of your own garden."
> **Nedra Glover Tawwab**

SELF-CARE – PRACTICE IT DAILY

Setting boundaries is essential for self-care and ensuring that your energy is spent on activities that bring value and joy to your life. Learning to say no to activities that drain your energy without offering any positive return is a crucial step towards self-care. This empowers you to prioritize what truly matters and engage in your favorite joyful activities. Apologies, ladies, but we often struggle the most when it comes to setting boundaries.

Be Clear and Direct:

- Communicate your limits clearly and assertively. Avoid ambiguous language that might lead to misunderstandings.
- Frame your boundaries with "I" statements to own your feelings and reduce defensiveness in others. For example, "I need some time to recharge this weekend, so I won't be able to join the outing."
- Although it might be difficult at first, practice saying no. Start with small refusals and gradually work up to bigger ones.

Areas of Your Life to Set Boundaries:

- Establish clear working hours and avoid taking work home. Learn to delegate tasks and say no to additional responsibilities that can overwhelm you.
- Set limits on how much time and energy you invest in toxic or draining relationships. Prioritize connections that uplift and support you.
- Limit your time on social media platforms to prevent them from consuming your day and affecting your mental health.
- Even with family, it's important to set boundaries. Assert your need for personal space and time without feeling guilty.

Setting boundaries is crucial to maintaining your mental, emotional, and physical health.

PASSION – DISCOVER AND IGNITE IT

Creating a vision board is a fun and engaging way to map out your goals and dreams. Think about some of your passions, long-term goals, and the emotions you want to experience.

Organize and Create Your Board:

- Start with a large piece of poster board or corkboard. Collect magazines, newspapers, printed images, scissors, glue, markers, and any other decorative items you might like.
- Dividing your board into sections helps to categorize your goals, such as personal growth, career, health, and relationships. This structure can make your vision more comprehensive.
- Flip through magazines and online resources to find images, words, and phrases that resonate with your goals and passions. Aim for visuals that evoke strong emotions and align internally.
- Include personal photos, quotes, or small trinkets that have special meaning to you. Personal touches can make your vision board more engaging and meaningful.
- Lay out your images and words on the board before gluing. Move them around until the arrangement feels right and then glue everything in place.

Utilizing Your Vision Board:

- Place your vision board in a spot where you will see it daily, such as your bedroom, office, or kitchen. Regularly viewing your board reinforces your goals and keeps you motivated.
- Spend a few minutes each day reflecting on your vision board. Visualize yourself achieving your goals and feeling the emotions associated with success.

Creating and regularly interacting with your vision board will provide clarity and inspiration, guiding you towards fulfilling your passions.

EAT AND ENJOY – NOURISHING FOOD

Maintaining proper hydration is essential for keeping your body nourished, sustaining energy levels, and supporting vital bodily functions.

Have you ever had a goldfish bowl? What happens to the fish when you don't change the water? The fish get sick and eventually die. Your body is 60-70% water, and your brain is almost 80% water! Think of your cells as the fish swimming in the "fishbowl of your body". If you don't refresh the water in your body daily by drinking enough water and consuming water-rich foods, the same thing that happened to the fish will happen to your cells—they will get sick and die.

Carry a Reusable Water Bottle:

- As a constant reminder to drink water, take a reuseable bottle with you.

Set Reminders:

- Use alarms on your phone as a reminder to drink water every hour. Divide your body weight in half, use this as a guide for how many ounces of water to drink daily.

Infuse Your Water:

- Add fresh fruits, herbs, or vegetables like cucumber, mint, or lemon.

Eat Water-Rich Foods:

- Incorporate water rich foods such as cucumbers, jicama, celery and melons. While living in Panama, I enjoyed jicama, a local vegetable sold on the street corners in a paper bag with fresh lime and sprinkle of salt. Enjoy the refreshing **Jicama and Tri-Colored Pepper Salad.**

Drink Before You're Thirsty:

- Don't wait until you're thirsty. Sip water throughout the day to maintain hydration.

Hydrating cells are happy cells and water helps keep you full.

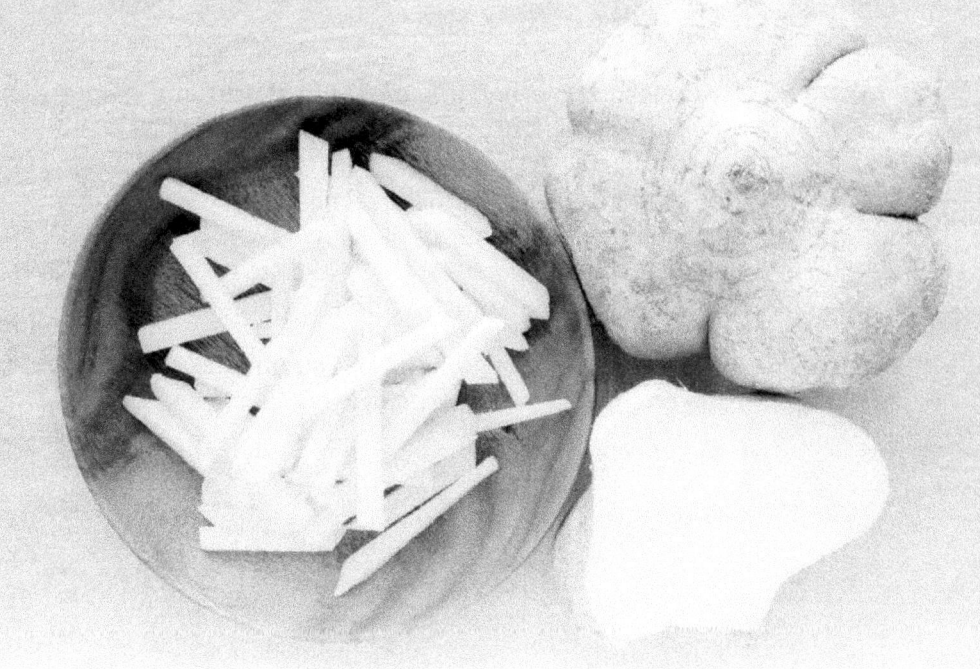

Jicama and Tri-Colored Pepper Salad

6 Servings

INGREDIENTS:

- ¼ cup lime juice
- 2 Tablespoons olive oil
- ½ teaspoon garlic powder
- ½ teaspoon cumin
- ½ teaspoon sea salt
- ½ red bell pepper, thinly sliced
- ½ yellow bell pepper, thinly sliced
- ½ orange bell pepper, thinly sliced
- ½ cup chopped red onion
- 1 large jicama (about 1 ½ lbs.), peeled and thinly sliced into matchsticks
- 1 cup cherry tomatoes, halved

PROCESS:

1. In large bowl, whisk together lime juice, olive oil, cumin, garlic powder and sea salt.

2. Add all veggies to bowl and toss well to coat with lime mixture.
3. Allow to sit for 30-60 minutes to mingle flavors and marinate.

With a water content of about 90%, jicama is packed with fiber and essential vitamins and minerals. It is low glycemic and low in calories, making it an ideal snack for those looking to manage their weight while still enjoying a crunchy, refreshing treat.

Use as a low-carb alternative to crackers: cut into slices and top with tuna, egg or chicken salad, or enjoy with hummus or dip.

ACTIVITY – EMBRACE AND LOVE MOVEMENT

Incorporating movement into your day doesn't have to be stressful. Start with getting up 5 times a day and performing 5 simple movements for 30 seconds each. That totals just 12.5 minutes a day! I put a sicky note on my computer that says, "You have 12.5 minutes, "Just do It!"

Jumping Jacks:

- Stand with your feet together and arms at your sides. Jump with your feet out while raising your arms above your head and then return to the starting position. For a modified version, rather than jumping, step your right leg out to the side while lifting your arms above your head. Repeat with your left leg.

High Knees:

- Stand tall and jog in place, bringing your knees up as high as possible with each step. Swing your arms to enhance the movement. Only raise knees as high as you are comfortable.

Squats:

- Stand with your feet shoulder-width apart and lower your body as if sitting back into a chair. Keep your chest up and knees behind your toes, then return to standing position.

Arm Circles:

- Extend your arms straight out to the sides at shoulder height and make small to large circular motions forward and backward.

Toe Touches:

- Stand with feet hip-width apart and keep your legs straight as you bend forward from the hips to touch your toes. Return to standing and repeat.

Always stay attuned to your body and mindful of any joint or back sensitivities.

KINDNESS – CULTIVATE IT IN YOUR DAILY LIFE

Forgiveness is a profound act of kindness that involves letting go of grudges and resentment towards others. By choosing to forgive, you release yourself from the heavy burden of anger and negativity, which can often weigh down your spirit and mental well-being.

Reflect and Understand:

- Take time to reflect on the situation and consider it from the other person's perspective. This can provide a comprehensive understanding of the situation, including their actions, fostering compassion, which is vital in the forgiveness process.

Express Your Feelings:

- Write a letter about your feelings towards the person or situation. Even if you don't send the letter; sometimes, just expressing your thoughts can be a crucial step toward forgiving. I recently started writing a forgiveness letter to an old friend and realized that forgiveness goes both ways; it's about asking for and offering it.

Seek Professional Help:

- Talking to a therapist or counselor can provide you with the tools and strategies to work through your feelings and move towards forgiveness in a healthy way. Some therapists offer group therapy sessions specifically focused on forgiveness.

Release Expectations:

- Let go of any expectations you have regarding apologies or reconciliation. Understand that forgiveness is a personal journey and is more about freeing yourself from negative emotions, regardless of the other person's actions.

By choosing to forgive, you empower yourself to live a more joyful and harmonious life.

Log Today's Activities and Experiences with The SPEAK Method

Use the questions or comments as a guide or write freely expressing your thoughts!

SELF-CARE – Where do you plan to set boundaries?

_____
_____
_____
_____
_____
_____
_____

PASSION – Draw out your vision board. What does it look like?

_____
_____
_____
_____
_____
_____
_____
_____

EAT AND ENJOY NOURISHING FOOD – How much water did you have today? What water rich vegetables are on your shopping list?

_____
_____
_____
_____
_____
_____
_____
_____

ACTIVITY – List the 5 movements you did for 30 seconds each.

_____
_____
_____
_____
_____
_____
_____
_____

KINDNESS – Who do you plan to forgive?

_____
_____
_____
_____
_____

ADDITIONAL NOTES

_____
_____
_____
_____
_____

DAILY REPORT CARD OF LIFE – How did you SPEAK today?

Grade Your Day, no D's or F's Allowed!

    A – Amazing

    B – Better than yesterday

    C – Challenging but working on it

Interview
Dr. Bridget Trammell, Doctorate in Christian Counseling, Business Coach, Certified Health Coach, and Public Speaker.

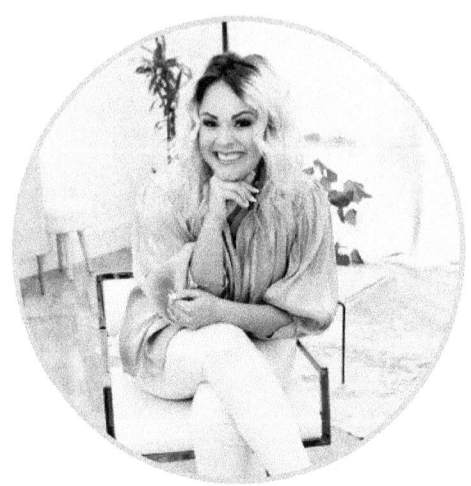

SELF-CARE – PRACTICE IT DAILY

Having six businesses, boundaries are extremely important, and the more influence you have the more boundaries you need. A boundary is not saying no, it is just saying yes to the greater need. Although we always put people over process, we maintain a culture of preserving our health so that burnout does not sabotage our goals.

PASSION – DISCOVER AND IGNITE IT

My passion has continued to evolve. After coaching over 8,000 clients to success with my health and wellness program, I found that not everyone that is depressed is sick, but most people who are sick are depressed. I began to uncover the stories of trauma behind the health problems, and this gave me a passion for mental health and healing. I eventually transitioned away from the weight loss industry to helping people heal their hearts.

EAT AND ENJOY - NOURISHING FOOD

With a husband and two active kids, I discovered that eating healthy doesn't have to be a full-time job. Both my husband and I have struggled with weight with our busy lifestyle. Keeping small, sustainable commitments has helped us gain success in small areas. For example, we don't keep sugar or white flour in our home, and we drink water with most meals. Making healthy choices doesn't have to be complicated!

ACTIVITY – EMBRACE AND LOVE MOVEMENT

With our children in elementary and middle school, our movements and activities involve the whole family! Walking the dog, taking a hike, or playing in the pool creates opportunities for exercise while sharing valuable family time.

KINDNESS – CULTIVATE IT IN YOUR DAILY LIFE

Kindness is the most important trait to teach our children, because without it, you cannot experience emotional healing. A child cannot self-regulate without a kind and caring adult, and many children grow into adults who have never experienced the repair of another human's attunement to their emotional state. The gift of kindness gives others around us the gift of healing, and we can then experience it ourselves. It is impossible to heal in the environment that made you sick. Pain is not a bad thing, but it can only be healed with kindness. Your influence only goes as far as your pain as deep, but kindness is the bridge that brings purpose to it.

<u>The Current Counseling Group</u>

DAY 8

"Nothing is impossible, the word itself says I'm possible"
Audrey Hepburn

SELF-CARE – PRACTICE IT DAILY

Positive affirmations are a powerful part of self-care because they help to reframe your mindset and foster a positive outlook on life. By consistently reinforcing positive thoughts, you can diminish negative self-talk and build self-confidence. This practice can lead to reduced stress, improved emotional health, and greater resilience in facing challenges.

I Am Worthy of Love and Respect:
- Take time each day to remind yourself of your positive qualities.
- Surround yourself with supportive and loving people.

Let Go of Negative Thoughts and Embrace Positivity:
- Engage in activities that promote a positive mindset, like reading uplifting books or listening to inspiring podcasts.
- Practice mindfulness or meditation to stay present and manage stress.

I Deserve Time to Myself to Relax and Recharge:
- Schedule downtime in your calendar and treat it as an important appointment.
- Indulge in activities that relax you, such as taking a bath, reading a book, or practicing a hobby.

I Can Achieve My Goals and Dreams:
- Break down your goals into manageable steps and celebrate small victories.
- Stay committed to your path, even when facing obstacles, and trust in your abilities.

I Choose to Focus on Things That Bring Me Joy and Fulfillment:
- Identify and prioritize activities and people that make you happy.
- Regularly reflect on what brings you joy and remove or minimize sources of stress.

Affirmations encourage you to concentrate on your strengths and potential.

PASSION – DISCOVER AND IGNITE IT

Making a list of your non-negotiables is vital for discovering and igniting your passion. These are the values, conditions, and aspects of work or life you won't compromise on. Knowing them helps you understand what you need to feel fulfilled and ensures you stay aligned with what truly makes you happy.

Throughout my life, I've encountered both significant successes and even greater failures. Having established and managed two brick-and-mortar businesses in the food service industry, I've realized that my current non-negotiable is steering clear of brick-and-mortar ventures!

Reflect on Past Experiences:

- Identify situations where you felt most fulfilled or drained. This helps clarify what you must have or avoid.

Assess Your Core Values:

- Determine the values that are central to your life. Knowing these can guide decisions and align actions with your passions.

Visualize Your Ideal Day:

- Imagine your perfect day from start to finish. The recurring themes or activities in your perfect day are likely non-negotiable.

Identify Deal-Breakers:

- List things that you know you absolutely cannot tolerate, whether it's in relationships, work environments, or life in general. My personal deal breakers are truth and integrity!

Evaluate Past Failures:

- Analyze situations where things didn't work out. Understanding what went wrong helps you identify what must be avoided in the future.

Identifying and adhering to your non-negotiables allows you create a foundation for a fulfilling and purpose-driven life.

EAT AND ENJOY – NOURISHING FOOD

Although not all sugar is evil, avoiding processed sugar is essential because it can lead to various health issues, such as obesity, heart disease, and Type 2 diabetes. Processed sugars can also impact mental health, leading to mood swings and decreased energy. By enjoying natural sweeteners, "You can have your cake and eat it too!"

Honey:

- Its natural antibacterial and antimicrobial properties enhance your immune system.
- Take teaspoon for sore throat, make honey butter, drizzle on a sweet potato or make cheesecake filling in the **Lemon Cheesecake and Fresh Fruit Parfaits.**

Maple Syrup:

- With a lower glycemic index than regular sugar, maple syrup has a milder impact on your blood sugar levels. It is also nutrient rich with potassium, iron, and zinc.
- Sweeten coffee, add to salad dressings, glaze meats and fish, add to plain yogurt, and enhance the flavor of sauces and gravies.

Monk Fruit:

- Revered by Buddhist monks, it is virtually calorie-free making it an excellent option for weight management. With a taste like traditional sugar, it is an easy replacement in recipes.
- Make homemade ice cream, sweeten lemonade, and use it in baked sweets.

Coconut Sugar:

- Contains inulin, a soluble fiber that can aid digestion, improve gut health, and potentially regulate blood sugar levels. The production of coconut sugar is more sustainable and environmentally friendly.
- Practical uses: As a substitute for brown sugar, use in recipes, sweeten oatmeal or make a tasty caramel.

Indulging in sweets is a delightful part of life, especially with these natural sweeteners.

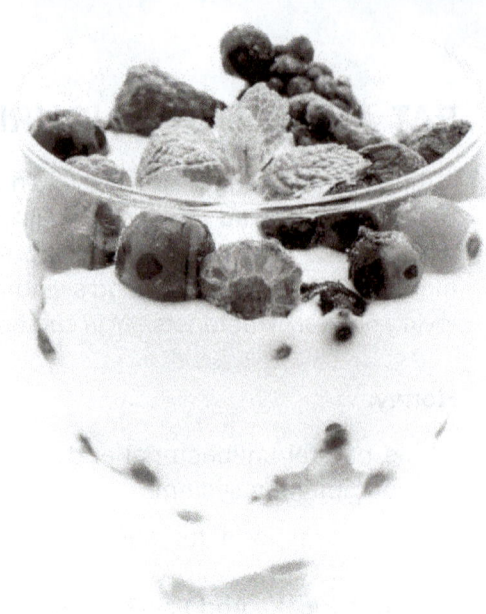

Lemon Cheesecake and Fresh Fruit Parfaits

6 Servings

INGREDIENTS:

- 1 - 8 oz. package low fat cream cheese, softened
- 3 Tablespoons honey
- 1/4 cup plain, non-fat Greek yogurt
- 1 lemon juiced and zested (save 1 Tablespoon for topping)
- 1 cup berries, a mixture of choice - strawberries, blueberries, raspberries, blackberries (Optional, mix with 1 teaspoon honey)

PROCESS:

1. In a medium bowl combine the cream cheese, honey, Greek yogurt, and lemon juice,
2. Using an electric mixer, blend at medium-high speed until smooth and creamy or use a spatula to mix until smooth.
3. Add zest and stir with a spatula or spoon.
4. Layer cream cheese mixture and berries, dividing ingredients equally. Top with additional lemon zest and serve!

ACTIVITY – EMBRACE AND LOVE MOVEMENT

Exploring museums, zoos, national or state parks, and historical sites can be a wonderful way to stay active while learning. Explore local attractions and plan day trips, weekend getaways, or vacations to enjoy them. My husband and I took an unforgettable journey through the Southwestern U.S., visiting Zion, Bryce Canyon, the Grand Canyon, Canyonlands, and Mesa Verde. It truly was the trip of a lifetime. Start planning your next getaway!

Museums:

- Participate in a guided tour that involves extra walking.
- Explore the museum's outdoor spaces or gardens to add variety and extra steps to your visit.

Historical Sites:

- Many towns offer guided walking tours through historic neighborhoods.
- Look for farm or agricultural tours that involve a lot of walking.
- My recent visit to Fort Pulaski National Monument, just outside of Savannah, GA, highlighted the region's rich military history and involved quite a bit of walking and climbing, including on an old Civil War cannon!

Zoos:

- Explore both large zoos and local farm animal interaction sites. I live near the Carl Sandburg home, where his wife was a renowned goat breeder. Running around with the baby goats in the spring is a fun and challenging way to stay active.
- Participate in interactive activities or training sessions.

National or State Parks:

- Choose more challenging or longer trails to get your heart rate up.
- Join guided nature walks to learn while you move.

With so much beauty in the world, it's time to get out and enjoy it.

KINDNESS – CULTIVATE IT IN YOUR DAILY LIFE

Visiting a new place can be an exciting adventure filled with exploration, discovery, and new experiences. By extending simple acts of kindness, rather than being the demanding tourist, you enrich your travel experience, foster deeper connections with the locals, and leave a positive impact on the community.

Engage in Conversations with locals:

- Compliment locals on their community by saying something like, "You are fortunate to live in such a wonderful place!"

Support Local Businesses:

- Shop and eat locally. Purchase souvenirs from local artisans and utilize local tour guides. This gives you a more authentic experience and supports the livelihood of those in the community.

Respect Cultural Norms and Practices:

- Understanding and respecting the local culture will create more meaningful interactions. Even within the United States, there are distinct cultural differences. My nieces, who grew up in Minnesota, embrace the local culture of friendliness known as "Minnesota Nice." One summer, while a niece from another state was visiting, they took her out on the lake in their pontoon boat. As they drifted along, they waved at everyone on the docks and in other boats. When asked if she knew those people, she replied, "No, we wave at everyone. It's just being 'Minnesota Nice.'"

Leave No Trace:

- Practice environmental kindness by minimizing your ecological footprint. Dispose of trash properly, use refillable water bottles, and respect wildlife and natural habitats.

No matter what state you live in, practice "Minnesota Nice," and we will have a happier country and world.

Log Today's Activities and Experiences with The SPEAK Method

Use the questions or comments as a guide or write freely expressing your thoughts!

SELF-CARE – List three positive affirmations.

_____
_____
_____
_____
_____
_____
_____

PASSION – List your non-negotiables for engaging in your passion.

_____
_____
_____
_____
_____
_____
_____

EAT AND ENJOY NOURISHING FOOD – What are your favorite healthy sweeteners? How do you plan on using them?

___

ACTIVITY – List local trips you want to take to attractions that will involve activity.

___

KINDNESS – Plan ahead on how you will practice kindness on your next trip.

_____
_____
_____
_____
_____
_____

ADDITIONAL NOTES

_____
_____
_____
_____
_____
_____

DAILY REPORT CARD OF LIFE – How did you SPEAK today?

Grade Your Day, no D's or F's Allowed!

- **A** – Amazing
- **B** – Better than yesterday
- **C** – Challenging but working on it

DAY 9

> "Food is not the problem, it's what we do with food that becomes the problem."
> **Joyce Meyer**

SELF-CARE – PRACTICE IT DAILY

Sleep is a fundamental part of self-care, providing essential restoration for both mind and body. Proper sleep fuels a healthier, happier life, allowing us to live with greater energy, positivity, and resilience. Adequate sleep helps your body to repair and rejuvenate, strength the immune system, and enhance cognitive function. Lack of sleep can lead to increased irritability, anxiety, and even depression.

Establish a Sleep Routine:

- Go to bed and wake up at the same time every day, even on weekends. This helps regulate your body's internal clock, improving sleep quality. Sticking to a consistent schedule can enhance your productivity and mood.

Create a Relaxing Bedtime Ritual:

- Engage in calming activities such as reading, meditating, or taking a warm bath before bed. Additionally, practicing gentle yoga is helpful. Avoid screens that emit blue light, which can interfere with your sleep cycle.

Mind Your Diet:

- Avoid caffeine, nicotine, and heavy meals close to bedtime. Instead, consider a light protein snack such as yogurt or a small handful of nuts. Additionally, herbal teas like chamomile can promote relaxation and help signal your body that it's time to wind down.

Optimize Your Sleep Environment:

- Keep your bedroom cool, dark, and quiet. Invest in a comfortable mattress and pillows and consider using blackout curtains or a white noise machine if necessary. Incorporating calming scents, such as lavender essential oil, can also create a serene environment conducive to restful sleep.

Prioritizing sleep is a vital step towards creating a balanced, fulfilling lifestyle.

PASSION – DISCOVER AND IGNITE IT

Embracing failures is an essential aspect of discovering and igniting your passion. Each setback provides invaluable lessons that help refine your path. Accept failures as stepping stones in the dynamic pursuit of your passion.

Learning Opportunities:

- Each failure provides invaluable lessons that can guide you towards better decisions in the future. By analyzing what went wrong, you can adapt and grow, making future attempts more successful.

Resilience Building:

- Facing failures builds mental and emotional resilience. The ability to bounce back from setbacks strengthens your determination and persistence, vital qualities when pursuing your passion.

I'm passionate about swimming in the ocean. My first boogie boarding attempt left me with a face full of sand and a cut leg from a rock. Despite the setbacks, I persisted and eventually enjoyed boogie boarding at Hilton Head Island for my 73rd birthday, injury-free.

Innovation and Creativity:

- Failures often force you to think outside the box and innovate. They push you to explore new perspectives and solutions, fostering creativity that can lead to breakthroughs in your passion.

Motivation Boost:

- Overcoming failures can be incredibly motivating. Each small victory after setback fuels your desire to keep going, reinforcing your commitment to your passion.

Encouraging Risk-Taking:

- Knowing that failure is a steppingstone to success encourages you to take calculated risks. This boldness is often necessary to make significant strides in your life goals.

Embracing failures ultimately transforms your journey of finding and igniting your passion.

EAT AND ENJOY – NOURISHING FOOD

Eating more whole foods and less processed food is essential for optimal health. Growing up in the 50's, it was rare that we ate processed foods, let alone what they now call ultra-processed. Now, Americans consume more than half of their daily calories as ultra-processed. A study published in *the British Medical Journal* found that people who consumed high amounts of these foods have an increased risk of anxiety, depression, obesity, metabolic syndrome and certain cancers. Eating and enjoying whole foods can be simple and affordable.

Start Simple:

- Begin by adding one whole food item to each meal, such as a piece of fruit, a serving of vegetables, or whole grains.

Whole Food Swaps:

- Substitute processed foods with whole food alternatives. For example, swap white rice with quinoa or brown rice and choose fresh fruit over sugary snacks.

Read Labels:

- When purchasing packaged items, choose products with minimal ingredients and avoid those with additives and preservatives.

Eat Seasonally:

- Choose fruits and vegetables that are in season. Seasonal produce is often fresher, more nutritious, and less expensive. Visit local farmers' markets to find seasonal whole foods.

Cook at Home:

- Preparing meals at home allows you to control ingredients and opt for whole food recipes. Experiment with new recipes that emphasize whole foods like vegetables, beans, and lean proteins.

Remember, if God made it, eat it, and if man made it, eat it in moderation or not at all!

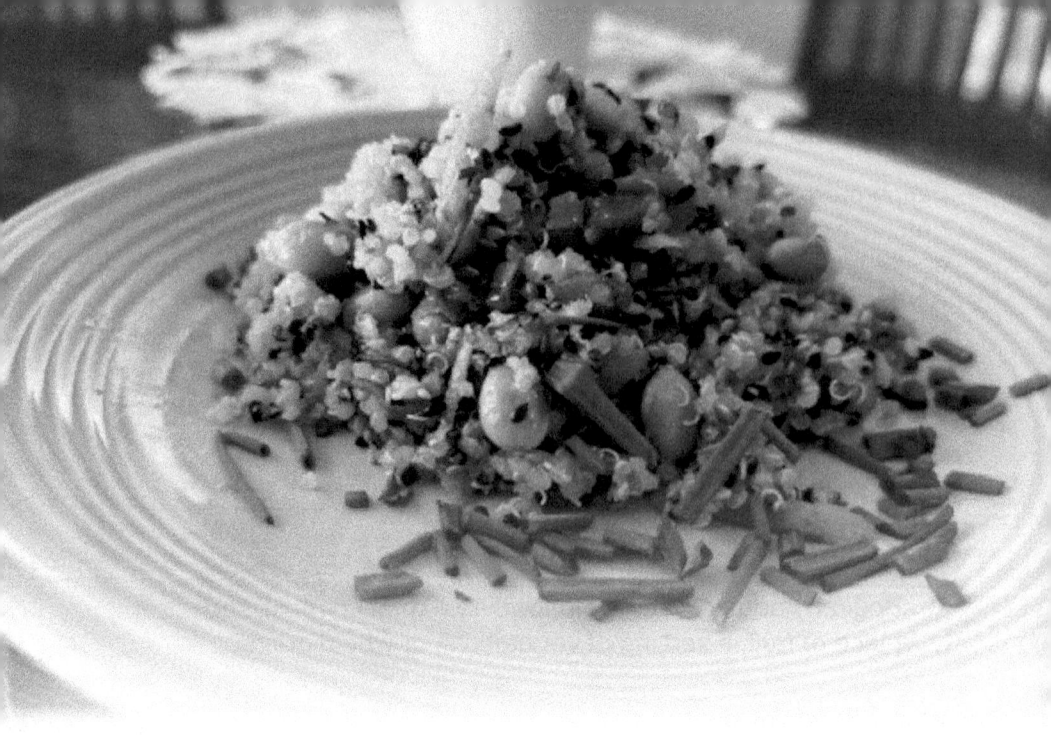

Asian Quinoa Salad

6 Servings

INGREDIENTS:

For the Salad:

- 1 cup quinoa, rinsed in fine sieve under cold water
- 2 cups water
- 1/4 teaspoon sea salt
- 1 cup shelled and cooked edamame or thawed frozen edamame
- 1 red bell pepper, chopped
- 1/2 cup shredded carrots
- 1 cup diced cucumber
- 2 Tablespoons chopped green onion

For the dressing:

- 1/4 cup lite soy sauce or tamari sauce low sodium
- 1 Tablespoon sesame oil
- 1 Tablespoon rice wine vinegar
- 1/4 cup chopped cilantro

- 1 Tablespoon sesame seeds
- 1/4 teaspoon grated ginger
- 1/8 teaspoon red pepper flakes
- Salt and black pepper to taste

PROCESS:

1. Add water, rinsed quinoa, and salt to a medium saucepan and bring to a boil over medium heat. Boil for 5 minutes. Turn the heat to low and simmer for about 15 minutes, or until water is absorbed. Remove from heat and fluff with a fork and allow to cool.
2. Place the quinoa in a large bowl and add the edamame, red pepper, carrots, green onions and cucumber. Set it aside.
3. In a small bowl, whisk together the soy sauce, sesame oil, rice wine vinegar, cilantro, sesame seeds, ginger, red pepper flakes, salt, and pepper.
4. Pour the dressing over the quinoa salad and stir to combine.
5. Top with optional toasted slivered or sliced almonds.

ACTIVITY – EMBRACE AND LOVE MOVEMENT

Whether you call it a shuffle, a waddle, or a penguin walk, moving on the balls of your feet engages your core and burns more calories. It's very similar to what boxers do when warming up in the ring. For over seven years, I've coached thousands of clients to integrate this movement, and those who adopted it experienced the most success in weight and inch loss. This low-impact exercise builds muscle, burns fat, can be performed at any age, and requires no special equipment—just your body.

How to Shuffle:

- Stand with feet should width apart.
- Roll up on your toes.
- Slightly bend your knees. (Never lock out your knees).
- Hold your core tight.
- Shuffle your feet side to side.
- Do not let your heals touch the ground.
- Start with alternating between walking or marching in place.

Where to Shuffle:

- Watching your favorite movie, TV series or while folding laundry.
- Listening to music, audio books or podcasts.
- Walking your dog. (Stop and shuffle when dog sniffs or does its "duties").
- Leisurely strolling the neighborhood. (Stop at crosswalks and shuffle).

A funny story: I had clients who, while strolling through their neighborhood, stopped at the crosswalk to shuffle. Another neighbor approached them to ask if they needed to use their bathroom, as it looked like the "potty dance." The good news is that now the whole neighborhood is shuffling together!

Embrace the joy and laughter of the penguin waddle, a delightful way to brighten your day.

KINDNESS – CULTIVATE IT IN YOUR DAILY LIFE

Active listening is crucial for practicing kindness, as it fosters understanding, strengthens relationships, and demonstrates genuine care. By listening attentively, we show respect and empathy, making others feel valued and heard. Remember, we have two ears and one mouth for a reason—listen more and talk less.

Improves Communication:

- Making eye contact shows you're genuinely absorbing their words and fully grasping the message. This minimizes misunderstandings and helps the person feel appreciated, thereby strengthening your connection.

Shows Engagement:

- Mirroring someone's body language can be an effective way to show you are truly engaged in the conversation. Subtly adopt similar postures, gestures, and facial expressions that the person you're speaking with is using. For instance, if they lean slightly forward and nod while talking, you can also lean forward and offer a nod when it feels natural.

Demonstrates Empathy:

- Place yourself in the speaker's shoes. This practice nurtures empathy, enabling you to grasp and share their emotions. Using phrases like "I completely understand," or "How did that make you feel" acknowledges and validates their feelings while demonstrating kindness and compassion.

Encourages Open Dialogue:

- Active listening fosters a safe space for honest dialogue, where individuals feel at ease expressing their true selves. This openness cultivates deeper, more authentic relationships and a greater sense of community and kindness. Use phrases such as "Tell me more" or "Explain what you mean."

Practicing active listening daily can profoundly enhance our interactions, showcasing genuine kindness and fostering stronger, more empathetic connections.

Log Today's Activities and Experiences with The SPEAK Method

Use the questions or comments as a guide or write freely expressing your thoughts!

SELF-CARE – What time are you going to bed and what are you going to do to prepare for a restful sleep?

_____
_____
_____
_____
_____
_____
_____

PASSION – List some of your failures and what you learned from them.

_____
_____
_____
_____
_____
_____
_____
_____
_____

EAT AND ENJOY – Create a shopping list of whole foods.

ACTIVITY – How many minutes did you shuffle? Are your calves burning yet?

KINDNESS – Who did you actively listen to today and what did you learn from it?

_____
_____
_____
_____
_____

ADDITIONAL NOTES

_____
_____
_____
_____
_____

DAILY REPORT CARD OF LIFE – How did you SPEAK today?

Grade Your Day, no D's or F's Allowed!

- **A** – Amazing
- **B** – Better than yesterday
- **C** – Challenging but working on it

DAY 10

"*I fear the day that technology will surpass our human interaction. The world will have a generation of idiots.*"
Albert Einstein

SELF-CARE – PRACTICE IT DAILY

Doing a digital detox is an excellent form of self-care that can help us reset and rejuvenate our mental and emotional well-being. In today's hyper-connected world, we're often inundated with information, notifications, and screen time, which can lead to stress, anxiety, and burnout. Excess screen time can also lead to eye stress.

Set Daily Screen Time Limits:

- Determine specific periods during the day when you allow yourself to use social media or browse the web. For example, you might allocate 30 minutes in the morning and another 30 minutes in the evening. Stick to these time slots to avoid mindless scrolling.

Use App Timers:

- Utilize built-in app timers like Screen Time on iOS or Digital Wellbeing on Android, or consider third-party apps like Moment or StayFocusd, to set specific limits on social media usage.

Create "No-Tech" Zones:

- Designate specific areas in your home where digital devices are prohibited to help foster more meaningful interactions and better rest. For example, make the dining room a tech-free zone to encourage family conversations during meals, and keep the bedroom device-free to promote better sleep hygiene.

Engage in Offline Activities:

- Engage in activities that don't involve screens to help refresh your mind and provide a break from digital distractions. Consider reading a captivating book, taking up painting, baking, or enjoying the great outdoors by taking a walk in nature.

Taking time to unplug is an act of self-care that provides lasting benefits for physical and mental health.

PASSION – DISCOVER AND IGNITE IT

Discovering your passion is a key step towards living a fulfilling and purpose-driven life. Taking personality tests can offer valuable insights into your interests, strengths, and motivations and are designed to help identify what truly excites and inspires you.

Identify Your Strengths and Interests:

- Start by taking tests that assess your strengths and interests, such as the CliftonStrengths assessment or the Myers-Briggs Type Indicator (MBTI). These tests can highlight your natural talents and preferences, guiding you towards activities and careers that align with your innate abilities and interests.

Reflect on Your Values and Motivations:

- Tests like the Values in Action (VIA) Survey can help you understand what drives you and what you value most in life. Knowing your core values can clarify which activities and goals resonate with your deeper sense of purpose.

Explore Career Matches:

- Consider taking career aptitude tests like the Strong Interest Inventory or the Holland Code (RIASEC) assessment. These tests match your interests and personality traits with potential career paths, offering suggestions that might align well with your passions.

Analyze Personality Traits:

- Personality tests, such as the Enneagram or the Big Five Personality Test, can provide insights into how your personality might influence your passions. Understanding your personality traits can help you identify the types of environments and activities where you are likely to thrive.

Embrace the journey of self-discovery and allow these tools to guide you towards a fulfilling personal life or career.

EAT AND ENJOY – NOURISHING FOOD

Fermented foods have been part of human diets for centuries. Known for their unique flavors, fermentation enhances nutritional value and digestibility, providing beneficial probiotics that support gut health.

Kimchi:

- This popular Korean dish, made from spicy fermented cabbage, is rich in vitamins and lactic acid bacteria, aiding digestion and boosting immunity. I am often reminded of my favorite TV series, "M*A*S*H," where they uncover buried pots of kimchi in the Korean battlefields.

Sauerkraut:

- This traditional fermented cabbage is packed with probiotics, which support gut health by balancing the gut microbiome. It's also high in vitamins C and K and contains anti-inflammatory properties, making it great for maintaining overall health.

Kefir and Yogurt:

- Both kefir and yogurt are fermented milk products rich in probiotics, calcium, and B vitamins. Kefir has a thinner consistency compared to yogurt, but both are high in probiotics to improve and boost the immune system. Try the **Greek Chicken Kebabs** recipe that incorporates yogurt in the marinade.

Miso:

- This traditional Japanese seasoning, made from fermented soybeans, is rich in essential minerals, B vitamins, and probiotics that support the immune system and gut health. Available as a paste or powder, it's commonly used to make the soup seen in Japanese restaurants.

Kombucha:

- A fermented beverage made from black tea, providing numerous health benefits with a slight effervescence.

Incorporating these fermented foods into your diet promotes a balanced gut and supports a healthy immune system.

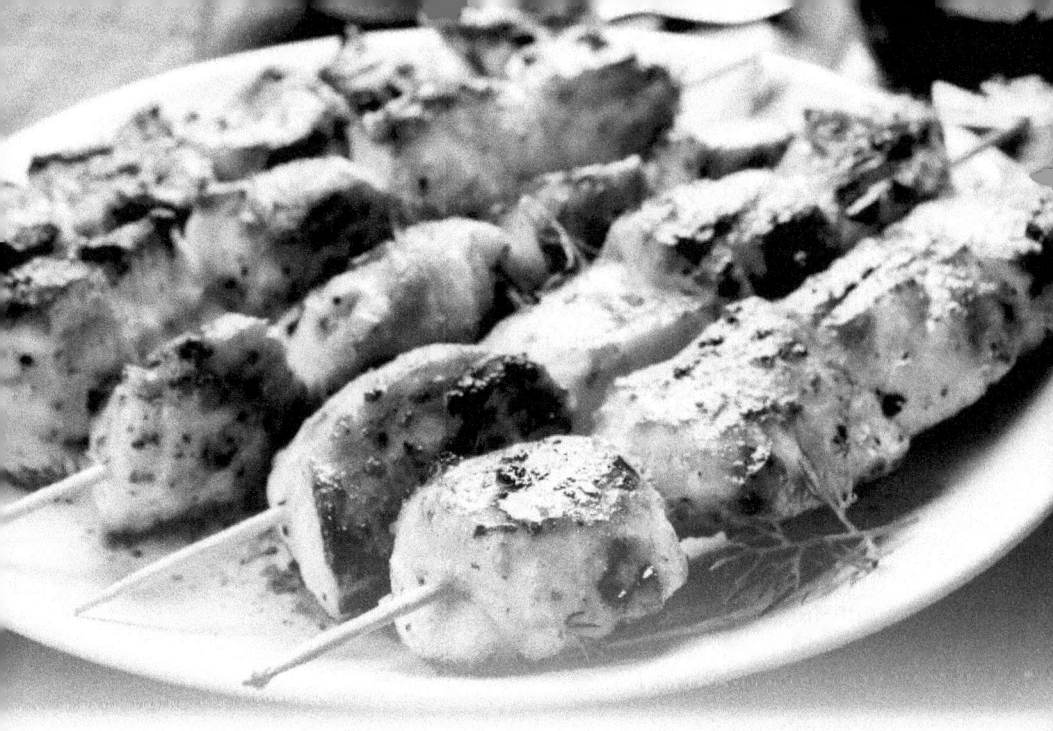

Greek Chicken Kebabs

6-8 Servings

INGREDIENTS:

- 1 cup plain whole milk Greek yogurt
- 3 Tablespoons olive oil
- 2 teaspoons paprika
- 1/2 teaspoon cumin
- 1/8 teaspoon cinnamon
- 1 teaspoon crushed red pepper flakes (reduce to 1/2 teaspoon if you don't like heat)
- Zest from one lemon
- 3 Tablespoons freshly squeezed lemon juice, from one lemon
- 1 teaspoon salt
- 1/2 teaspoon freshly ground black pepper
- 4 garlic cloves, minced
- 2-1/2 pounds boneless skinless chicken thighs (or 2 pounds boneless skinless chicken breasts), trimmed of any excess fat and cut into large bite-sized pieces
- 1 large red onion, cut into wedges

PROCESS:

1. In a medium bowl, combine the yogurt, olive oil, paprika, cumin, cinnamon, red pepper flakes, lemon zest, lemon juice, salt, pepper and garlic.

2. Thread the chicken onto metal skewers, folding if the pieces are long and thin, alternating occasionally with the red onions. Note: You'll need between 6-8 skewers.)

3. Place the kebabs on a baking sheet lined with aluminum foil. Spoon or brush the marinade all over the meat, coating well. Cover and refrigerate at least eight hours or overnight.

4. Preheat the grill to medium-high heat. To grease the grill, lightly dip a wad of paper towels in vegetable oil and, using tongs, carefully rub over the grates several times until glossy and coated.

5. Grill the chicken kebabs until golden brown and cooked through, turning skewers occasionally, 10 to 15 minutes.

ACTIVITY – EMBRACE AND LOVE MOVEMENT

It may sound silly, but tapping your feet while at your desk or any chair is a discreet and simple way to incorporate movement into your day. By regularly tapping your feet, you boost blood flow to your lower extremities, engage muscles, and enhance overall energy levels and focus. This effortless movement can break the monotony of prolonged sitting, promoting better posture and reducing the risk of developing sedentary-related health issues, including blood clots. Be sure to engage the core while foot tapping. I almost wore a hole in floor from all the foot tapping while writing this book!

Heel-Toe Taps:

- Sit up straight with your feet flat on the floor.
- Tap your heels against the floor, followed by your toes.
- Repeat, ensuring movements are rhythmic and steady.

Alternating Foot Taps:

- Keep your back straight and feet flat.
- Lift your right foot slightly off the floor and tap it down lightly.
- As you put your right foot down, lift your left foot and repeat the tap.

Double Foot Taps:

- Sit with both feet flat on the floor.
- Simultaneously tap both feet on the floor, lifting them just an inch or two.
- Maintain a steady rhythm.

Side-to-Side Taps:

- Sit comfortably with your feet flat.
- Slowly move both feet from side to side, tapping the outer edge of your right foot.
- Return to the center and then tap the outer edge of your left foot.

Foot tapping can be easily incorporated into your daily routine without disrupting your workflow.

KINDNESS – CULTIVATE IT IN YOUR DAILY LIFE

The age-old American proverb, "A smile is worth a thousand words," emphasizes the power of a simple smile to spread kindness and positivity. A smile can quickly forge connections and brighten someone's day.

Meeting New People:

- A smile creates an immediate connection, making introductions more pleasant and easing any initial tension. Smiling can make you appear more approachable, trustworthy, and warm, which can set the tone for positive interaction and new relationships.

During a Disagreement:

- Smiling can help diffuse a heated situation, showing that you're open to finding a compromise and fostering a more constructive dialogue. In moments of conflict, a smile indicates that you are not approaching the situation with hostility and are willing to listen.

Customer Service Interactions:

- Whether you're the customer or the service provider, a smile encourages a positive and friendly exchange. It sets a positive tone and fosters an environment of mutual respect.

    My husband has the lovely habit of complimenting customer service representatives on their beautiful smiles, which always makes them beam with joy. He follows up by saying, "Thank you for being you!"

When Giving Feedback:

- Smiling while offering constructive criticism can help soften the message, making the recipient more receptive and less defensive. By smiling, you show that your intentions are positive and that you care about the person's growth and improvement.

Make it a habit to smile at everyone you meet – whether they are friends, colleagues, or strangers.

Log Today's Activities and Experiences with The SPEAK Method

Use the questions or comments as a guide or write freely expressing your thoughts!

SELF-CARE – How many minutes were you on a screen today? How are you going to limit screen time?

_____
_____
_____
_____
_____
_____

PASSION – List personality tests you explored or ones you plan to explore.

_____
_____
_____
_____
_____
_____
_____
_____

EAT AND ENJOY NOURISHING FOOD – What fermented foods do you have on hand and list ones for your shopping list?

_____
_____
_____
_____
_____
_____
_____
_____

ACTIVITY – List the tapping movements you tried.

_____
_____
_____
_____
_____
_____
_____
_____

KINDNESS – Who did you smile at today?

_____
_____
_____
_____
_____
_____

ADDITIONAL NOTES

_____
_____
_____
_____
_____
_____

DAILY REPORT CARD OF LIFE – How did you SPEAK today?

Grade Your Day, no D's or F's Allowed!

- **A** – Amazing
- **B** – Better than yesterday
- **C** – Challenging but working on it

DAY 11

"What I have learned for myself is that I don't have to be anybody else. Myself is good enough."
Lupita Nyong'o

SELF-CARE – PRACTICE IT DAILY

I'm not certain who first coined the phrase "the grass is greener on the other side," but it doesn't really matter. Everyone has struggles; they just may be different from yours. In a social media-driven society that constantly pushes us to compare ourselves to others, it's easy to feel inferior.

Set Personal Goals:

- Focus on your own growth and development by setting personal goals that are meaningful to you. Celebrate each achievement, no matter how small, to maintain momentum and a positive outlook.

Practice Self-Compassion:

- Be kind to yourself. Understand that it's okay to have flaws and make mistakes. Treat yourself with the same understanding and kindness you would offer a friend. This nurturing attitude can boost your resilience and overall well-being, fostering a healthier relationship with yourself.

Limit Social Media Use:

- Reduce the time you spend on social media platforms that often encourage comparison. Use that time to engage in activities that bring you fulfillment and joy. Whether it's reading a book, taking a walk, or pursuing a hobby, prioritize experiences that enrich your life and nurture your spirit.

Surround Yourself with Positivity:

- Spend time with uplifting people who inspire and support you. Engage in positive environments that reinforce your self-worth and individuality. I follow the motto "Positivity breeds positivity and negativity breeds negativity." When given the choice, who do you want to spend time with?

Remember that your cup is always half full, not half empty; celebrate the amazing person you are!

PASSION – DISCOVER AND IGNITE IT

Identifying patterns in your life is a powerful way to uncover or ignite your passion. By recognizing recurring themes, behaviors, and interests, you can gain valuable insights into what truly excites and motivates you.

Reflect on Past Experiences:

- Take time to think back on moments when you felt genuinely happy and fulfilled. What were you doing? Who were you with? What was the setting? Identifying common factors in these experiences can reveal underlying passions that you might not have fully recognized before.

Examine Your Reading and Media Preferences:

- Look at the types of books, articles, podcasts, and movies you gravitate towards. Your preferences in the media can often reflect your underlying interests and passions. One of my favorite books is "Under the Tuscan Sun." It incorporates travel, adventure, and cooking—my three passions.

Review Your Career and Education Choices:

- Examine the choices you've made in your career and education. Consider the subjects you studied, the roles you've excelled in, and the projects you loved working on. These decisions can provide clues about your true interests and desires.

Recognize and Address Negative Patterns:

- Identifying and understanding negative patterns in your behavior or thought processes is crucial. Once recognized, you can take conscious steps to alter these patterns, paving the way for personal growth and a clearer path to your true passions.

Understanding these patterns in your life will help focus your energy on pursuits that bring you joy and fulfillment.

EAT AND ENJOY – NOURISHING FOOD

Sometimes, we simply don't have time to cook or need to grab something quick. Opt for healthy snack meals by combining lean proteins with fresh fruits, vegetables, whole grains, and healthy fats. By keeping these nutritious items on hand, you're less likely to reach for that bag of chips, candy bar, or sugar-laden granola bar.

Greek Yogurt Parfait:
- Layer Greek yogurt with low or no sugar granola, fresh berries, and a sprinkle of walnuts.

Apple Slices with Almond or Peanut Butter:
- Dip apple slices in almond or peanut butter and a drizzle of honey.

Tuna or Chicken Salad on Whole Grain Crackers:
- Mix tuna or chicken with Greek yogurt, diced celery, and serve atop whole grain crackers.

Cottage Cheese and Fruit:
- Pair cottage cheese with fresh pineapple or cantaloupe chunks and a sprinkle of pumpkin seeds.

Turkey and Avocado Roll-Ups:
- Wrap turkey slices around avocado slices and cherry tomatoes.

Make a Simple Smoothie:
- Blend frozen berries, spinach, Greek yogurt and a scoop of plant-based protein powder for a nutrient-rich smoothie.

Avocado Toast:
- Top whole grain toast with mashed avocado, a poached or fried egg, and a sprinkle of sunflower seeds.

Make Homemade Granola Bars:
- Try the **Chocolate Granola Bars** with nuts, whole grains, and a touch of maple syrup.

The key to healthy snacks is to make them feel substantial, ensuring you won't overeat at your next meal.

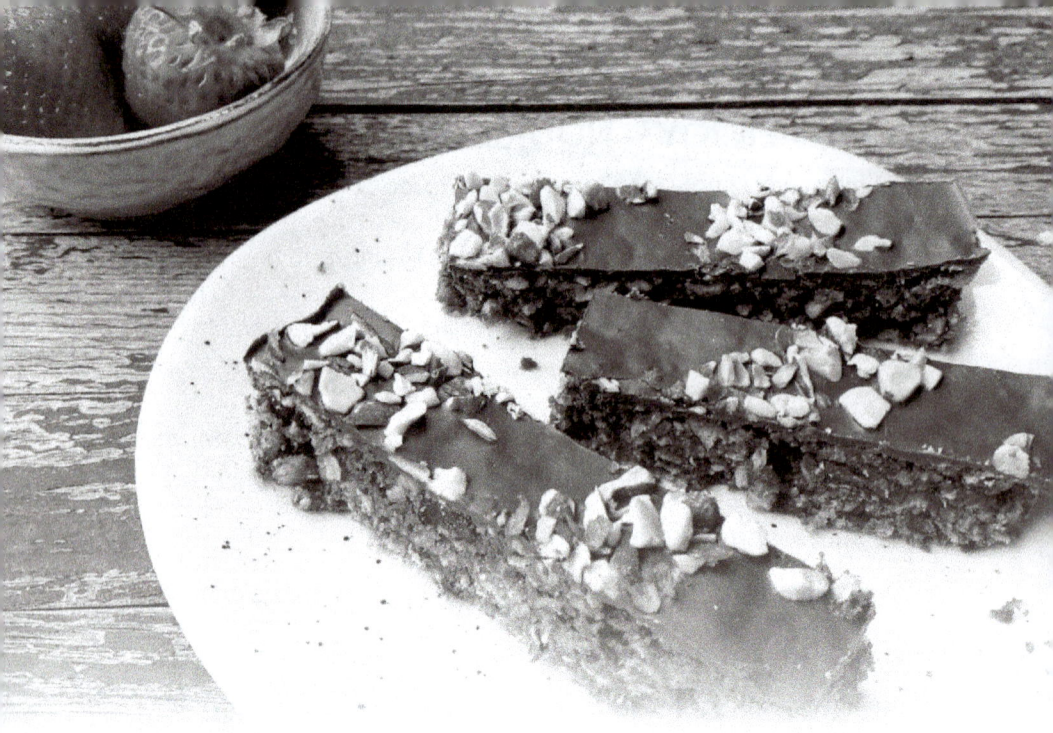

Chocolate Granola Bars

Serves 10-12

INGREDIENTS:

- 1/4 cup coconut oil
- 1 cup almond butter
- ½ cup maple syrup
- ½ cup almond milk
- 1 teaspoon vanilla
- 2 ½ cups rolled oats
- 1 cup brown rice cereal (One Degree Organic)
- ½ cup slivered or sliced almonds
- ½ cup dark chocolate chips (low or sugar-free)

Chocolate Nut Topping:

- 1/4 cup dark chocolate chips (low or sugar-free)
- 1/2 Teaspoon coconut oil
- 1/4 cup chopped almonds

Melt chocolate and coconut oil in microwave at 10 second intervals, stirring until smooth.

PROCESS:

1. Preheat oven to 325°F and line an 9X9 dish with parchment paper.
2. Melt coconut oil over low heat, add almond butter, almond milk, maple syrup, and vanilla. Stir until smooth and remove from heat.
3. In a separate bowl combine your dry ingredients (oats, rice cereal, almonds, and chocolate). Mix well.
4. Add the dry ingredients to wet ingredients and combine.
5. Transfer to baking dish and firmly press down to evenly spread into one smooth layer.
6. Bake 20 minutes and allow to cool for 10 minutes.
7. Top with melted dark chocolate and chopped almonds!
8. Cool for 30 minutes in refrigerator before cutting!

ACTIVITY – EMBRACE AND LOVE MOVEMENT

Some days, you just don't have time for designated exercise. On those days, ensure your NEAT is high. NEAT (Non-Exercise Activity Thermogenesis) may sound complex, but it simply means the energy expended during everyday activities that aren't formal exercise. If your job or day is sedentary, your NEAT is low; if it involves a lot of movement, your NEAT is high.

Increasing your NEAT can be a game-changer for maintaining an active lifestyle. Every little bit of movement counts and accumulates to enhance your overall energy expenditure.

NEAT ACTIVITIES:

- Walking while on phone calls.
- Taking the stairs instead of the elevator.
- Gardening or yard work.
- House cleaning or tidying up.
- Playing with children or pets.
- Cooking and meal preparation rather than take out.
- Fidgeting, tapping foot or pacing.
- Running errands on foot or by bike.
- Using a standing desk.
- Doing light stretching during breaks.

While writing this book, I made it a point to frequently get up, play with my dog or take her on walks to the mailbox to keep myself moving. On top of that, I intentionally chose a smaller water bottle so I would have to make more trips to the kitchen to refill it. These small, deliberate actions not only gave me mental breaks but also helped incorporate more physical activity into my day.

These small actions will help you stay active, even without a formal workout.

KINDNESS – CULTIVATE IT IN YOUR DAILY LIFE

Recommending a good book, podcast, or movie to a friend can be a thoughtful act of kindness that fosters connection and enriches their life. Here are four of my favorite shares.

A Thought-Provoking Book:

- One of my favorite thought-provoking books is "Atomic Habits" by James Clear. It offers actionable guidance on how small, daily habits lead to substantial improvements over time, making it an invaluable resource for enhancing both personal and professional development.

An Engaging Podcast:

- The podcast "On Being" with Krista Tippett, known for its tagline "Conversations to Live By," explores a wide array of topics, including spirituality, science, and social issues. This podcast can inspire introspection and expand one's understanding of the world.

An Uplifting Movie:

- The inspirational film, "The Pursuit of Happiness" provides motivation and hope. It is the true story of Chris Gardner's journey from homelessness to success and shows the power of perseverance and the importance of never giving up on one's dreams.

A Relaxing Show:

- One of my favorites is "Chef's Table", a visually stunning and relaxing show that offers a chance to unwind and enjoy captivating storytelling. This original series, produced by Netflix, explores the lives of world-renowned chefs, showcasing their creativity and passion for food.

By sharing your own recommendations, you're not only sharing a piece of what you enjoy but also enriching your friend's life with new experiences and insights.

Log Today's Activities and Experiences with The SPEAK Method

Use the questions or comments as a guide or write freely expressing your thoughts!

SELF-CARE – List ways you celebrated yourself today.

_____
_____
_____
_____
_____
_____
_____

PASSION – What patterns have you identified?

_____
_____
_____
_____
_____
_____
_____

EAT AND ENJOY NOURISHING FOOD – List your favorite snack meals and how you will make them healthy.

_____
_____
_____
_____
_____
_____
_____
_____
_____

ACTIVITY – Rate your NEAT (Non-Exercise Activity Thermogenesis). Is it high or low?

_____
_____
_____
_____
_____
_____
_____
_____
_____

KINDNESS – List enjoyable things you want to share with friends. What friends are you excited to share these with?

_____
_____
_____
_____
_____

ADDITIONAL NOTES

_____
_____
_____
_____
_____
_____

DAILY REPORT CARD OF LIFE – How did you SPEAK today?

Grade Your Day, no D's or F's Allowed!

- **A** – Amazing
- **B** – Better than yesterday
- **C** – Challenging but working on it

Interview
Lynda Sloan, B.F.A, M.A.
Psychospiritual Therapist, Artist

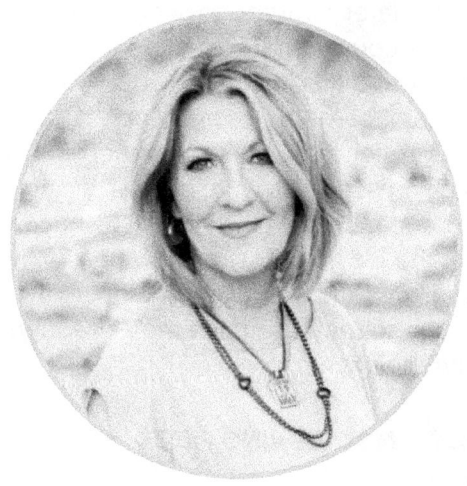

SELF-CARE – PRACTICE IT DAILY

I woke up one morning at 17 years of age with excruciating back pain. After five years of pain, consulting with 10 doctors and an exploratory surgery, I realized I needed to take charge of my own health. I stepped into a new world of "holistic health" incorporating chiropractic care, applied kinesiology, yoga, spirituality, and clean eating. I am so grateful I had the awakening to do this and I have never looked back. Over time I realized that how I start my morning sets the tone for the rest of my day. I pray, meditate and stretch, often before I even get out of bed. The simple task of making my bed starts the active part of my day. I am not a breakfast eater and have found that eating between 10am and 6pm works the best for my system. I try to do some activity each day like walking, pickleball or light weights, and something to keep my creative juices alive!

PASSION – DISCOVER AND IGNITE IT

Creating and surrounding myself with beauty is my passion. I entered college knowing I did not want to be a nurse or a teacher so I chose art as a major. I started working for homebuilders decorating their model homes and was able to transfer my artistic ability to interior design. I later returned to school for a graduate degree in psychology and counseling because I wanted to help others live a better life. Around this time Feng Shui was just coming to the west. Working a dual career of therapy and design I realized that our living spaces reflect our personal inner landscape and vice versa. As both an artist and psychospiritual therapist, my goal is to help people understand how their" interior spaces" can be redesigned to attract the life they desire. True beauty, not commercialized beauty is high vibration. I teach my clients how to discern high from low vibrations so they can raise their "frequency" and attract more beauty into their lives.

EAT AND ENJOY – NOURISHING FOOD

My mother was a stay-at-home mom and a great cook. Dinner was put in front of me every night so I did not think much about food until I started healing my back issue and was living on my own in my twenties. I turned to yoga as part of my healing modality, and at that time, studying Hinduism and being a vegetarian were part of this path. I can remember going to the grocery store in the late 70's and awakening to the fact that over 90% of what was in there was not whole or living food. I just assumed future generations would gravitate to healing and healthy eating as I did. While this isn't always the case, I am grateful that I was able to pass on to my family the understanding that food can be joyful but also "medicine". As a single mom on the go, I learned to be creative with ingredients. I did not have a lot of time to plan and shop but I learned that if I bought whole fresh foods, spices, and had beans and grains on hand I could make a variety of meals. I believe presentation is important and should be appealing to the palette. Healthy eating is more than just the ingredients it is also the energy you put into it – the consciousness, thoughts and feelings.

ACTIVITY – EMBRACE AND LOVE MOVEMENT

I have never been a "sitter", I think I would have been diagnosed as having ADHD if they had had that when I was younger. My mother said I would never sit still. When I personally think of *activity* I think of the Sun and being outside. The Sun is like a battery charger for me, which is why I chose to live in Arizona most of the year! I enjoy walking, hiking, racquet sports, and just being outside in nature. It saddens me that our culture is programming young people to be more sedentary and that obesity is acceptable and taking pharmaceuticals is okay. Movement of any kind is so important, movement IS life!

KINDNESS – CULTIVATE IT IN YOUR DAILY LIFE

I believe the way to cultivate kindness in one's life is to start by being kind to yourself and those that are closest to you. We are often our own worst enemy and rarely slow down to listen to the negative and critical voices in our head. These often reveal themselves in our relationships. Kindness, to me, refers to the gestures, thoughts and feelings of having an "open heart"; of accepting and allowing other's differences. I often refer to the heart as the "female brain". How would our life be different if we allowed her to guide us?

Radiant Light Studio

lynda@radiantlightstudio.com

DAY 12

"There is a fountain of youth: it is your mind, your talents, the creativity you bring to your life and the lives of people you love. When you learn to tap this source, you will truly have defeated age."
Sophia Loren

SELF-CARE – PRACTICE IT DAILY

Feeling younger goes beyond just maintaining physical health; it's about nurturing a youthful spirit as well. Embracing childlike behaviors can bring joy and energy into our lives, sparking creativity and positivity. Always remember to laugh with the carefree joy of a child.

Play Without Purpose:

- Set aside time to engage in playful activities simply for the sake of having fun. Jump on a swing, play board games, or build something with LEGO's. My niece Riley took up LEGO's in her 20's and has created artistic masterpieces from Disney castles to beautiful flowers.

Embrace Curiosity:

- Children are naturally curious and eager to learn. Approach the world with a sense of wonder and ask questions about things you don't know. This curiosity opens doors to new experiences and will enrich your journey in unexpected ways.

Be Present:

- Children live in the moment and find joy in the present. Practice mindfulness by noticing the world around you, savoring your meals, and being fully engaged in conversations. Being present can help you appreciate the small moments of life and feel younger at heart.

Create and Imagine:

- Take time to let your imagination run wild. Write a whimsical story, paint a picture, or daydream about fantastical worlds. Creative expression will keep your mind sharp, foster innovation and help you see the world from fresh, inspiring perspectives.

Incorporating these behaviors into your daily life will not only make you feel younger but also improve your emotional health and cultivate a positive outlook.

PASSION – DISCOVER AND IGNITE IT

Identifying and igniting your passion is a journey that can be greatly enhanced by speaking with various professionals who offer unique perspectives and expertise.

Career Coaches:

- Career coaches specialize in helping individuals discover their professional interests and strengths. They can provide personalized assessments, exercises, and guidance to help you identify what truly excites you. Their experience in aligning your skills with potential career paths can be invaluable in finding your passion.

Industry Experts:

- Speaking with professionals who are already established in a field that interests you can offer practical insights that are difficult to find elsewhere. They can share their personal experiences, the challenges they face, and the rewards of their work. This realistic view can either solidify your interest or help you refine your focus.

Entrepreneurs:

- Entrepreneurs are often driven by passion and innovation. Interviewing them can reveal how they turned their interests into viable businesses. They can provide advice on overcoming obstacles, staying motivated, and the importance of resilience. Their stories of following their dreams can be incredibly motivating.

Mentors or Advisors:

- Individuals who have served as mentors or advisors can offer long-term perspectives and wisdom. They typically possess a wealth of experience and have often guided others in discovering their passions. Their insights can help you navigate your own journey with a clearer vision and strategic approach.

Remember, the journey is unique for everyone, and talking to those who have walked the path before you can be enlightening and inspiring.

EAT AND ENJOY – NOURISHING FOOD

One-pot meals simplify cooking by combining all ingredients in a single pot, making preparation and cleanup a breeze. These delicious hearty dishes are perfect for busy lifestyles and allow for balanced nutrition with proteins, vegetables, and grains.

Stews:

- Hearty and comforting, stews typically combine meat, vegetables, and broth, simmered together until tender. Examples include beef stew, chicken stew, or a vegetarian lentil stew.

Casseroles:

- These oven-baked dishes often combine protein, vegetables, pasta, rice, or grains with a sauce or cheese, cooked together in one pot or dish. Try an old-fashioned tuna noodle casserole or my client's favorite **Cheeseburger Casserole.**

Curries:

- Rich and flavorful, curries often feature meat or vegetables simmered in a spiced sauce, typically served with rice or bread. Try chicken curry, vegetable curry, or Thai green curry.

One Pan Stir-fry:

- Quick and versatile, stir-frying involves cooking protein and vegetables in a single pan or wok with a sauce. Serve over rice or noodles. Try Mongolian beef stir-fry, sesame tofu stir-fry, or Kung Pao shrimp stir-fry.

Paella:

- A Spanish rice dish typically cooked in a single large pan, combining rice, saffron, vegetables, and a variety of proteins like seafood, chicken, or sausage. Try traditional Paella Valenciana.

Expand your one-pot meal repertoire by utilizing crockpots or Instant Pots.

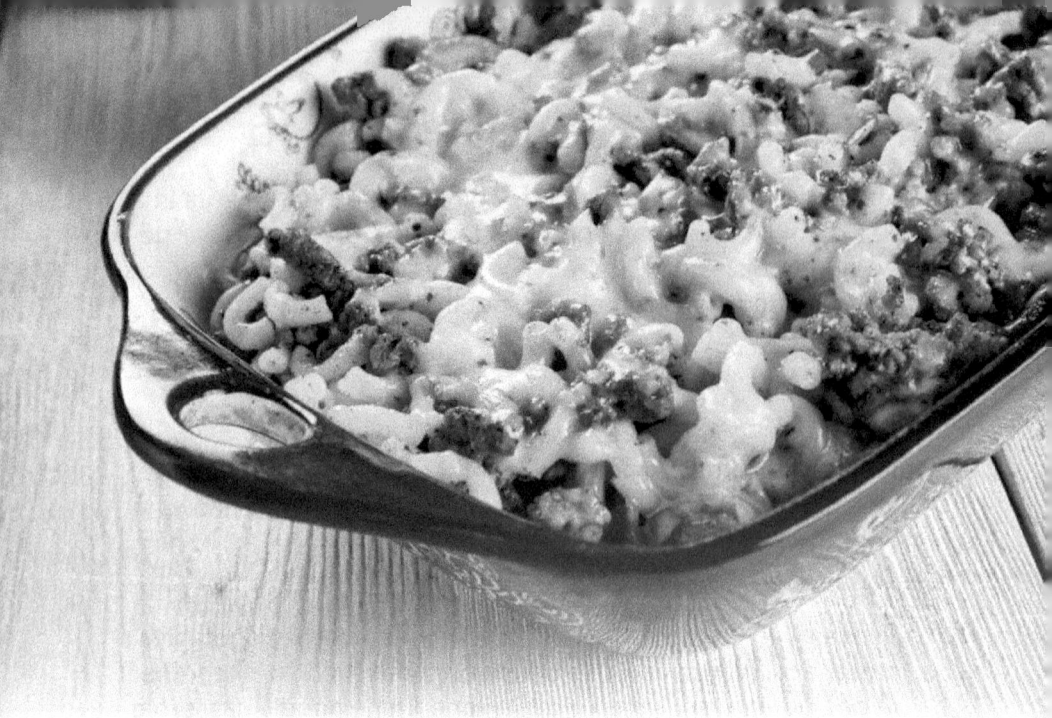

Cheeseburger Casserole

6 Servings

INGREDIENTS:

- 8 oz. whole-wheat or gluten free elbow macaroni
- 3 Tablespoons olive oil
- 1/2 cup onion, minced
- 1 Tablespoon garlic, minced
- 1 lb. ground lean ground meat (turkey, chicken or beef)
- 1/2 teaspoon paprika
- ½ teaspoon sea salt
- ¼ teaspoon black pepper
- 1 Tablespoon Italian seasoning
- 1 1/4 cup shredded sharp cheddar cheese
- 6 oz. low fat cream cheese
- 1/2 cup chicken broth
- Optional to add extra nutrition: 4 cups chopped spinach

PROCESS:

1. Preheat the oven to 350°F.

2. Oil a 9x13 casserole dish.
3. Bring a large pot of water to a boil, add pasta, and cook until al dente.
4. Drain in colander and rinse under cold water then toss with 1 Tablespoon olive oil.
5. Heat 2 Tablespoons olive oil in a large skillet over medium heat until shimmery.
6. Add onion and garlic and sauté, stirring until onion is translucent.
7. Add ground meat and spices. Cook, stirring frequently, until the meat is no longer pink. Drain off any excess juices and return to pan.
8. Add the cream cheese and chicken broth to the pan and heat on low to incorporate.
9. Remove from heat, put in bowl with the drained pasta add 1 cup shredded cheese, optional chopped spinach and mix well.
10. Put in oiled casserole dish and top with 1/4 cup shredded cheese.
11. Bake until the cheese is melted and the mixture bubbles, 20 to 25 minutes.

ACTIVITY – EMBRACE AND LOVE MOVEMENT

Strengthen your lungs with deep breathing exercises. These can significantly enhance your well-being by improving lung function and capacity.

Diaphragmatic Breathing:

- This method involves breathing deeply into your diaphragm rather than your chest. Sit or lay down in a comfortable position. Place one hand on your chest and the other on your belly. Inhale slowly through your nose, allowing abdomen to rise while the chest remains still. Exhale gently through your mouth. Benefits: Strengthens diaphragm and improves lung efficiency.

4-7-8 Breathing:

- Begin by inhaling quietly through your nose for 4 seconds. Hold your breath for 7 seconds, then exhale completely through your mouth for 8 seconds. Repeat this cycle several times. The 4-7-8 method can help to regulate your breathing pattern and reduce anxiety. Benefits: Helps regulate breathing pattern and reduces anxiety.

Pursed-Lip Breathing:

- This technique is especially beneficial for individuals with respiratory issues. Inhale slowly through your nose, then exhale through pursed lips, as if you were blowing out a candle. Exhale for twice as long as you inhaled. Benefits: Keeps airways open longer and reduces shortness of breath.

Box Breathing:

- This method involves breathing in a structured pattern to enhance focus and lung capacity. Inhale through your nose for 4 seconds, hold your breath for 4 seconds, exhale through your mouth for 4 seconds, and then hold your breath for another 4 seconds. Repeat several times. Benefits: Boost lung function and improve mental clarity.

Incorporate these daily habits to maintain lung health and mental clarity.

KINDNESS – CULTIVATE IT IN YOUR DAILY LIFE

In today's digital age, the charm and significance of handwritten cards or postcards often get overshadowed by the convenience of social media and texting. However, taking the time to write a heartfelt note shows a unique thoughtfulness.

Personal Touch:

- Instead of simply writing "thinking of you," take the time to craft a unique message: "Thought of you when hiking and remembered our great Colorado hikes together." Your personalized message will show the special bond you share. Pick a card with a picture that reminds you of the person.

Celebrating Milestones:

- A handwritten card to celebrate a birthday, anniversary, or retirement can add a personal touch that a digital message may lack. Congratulate a friend on their retirement with a card that includes a message about enjoying the next chapter of their life. Choose a colorful, fun and vibrant card.

Offering Support:

- Sending a comforting card to a friend or family member going through a tough time shows empathy and support. A handwritten sympathy card for someone who has lost a loved one lets them know you're there for them. Choose a card with calming scenes.

Expressing Gratitude:

- A thank-you card, after receiving a thoughtful gift or for someone's kindness, leaves a lasting impression. Sending a handwritten note thanking someone for hosting a memorable dinner party or for simply being a supportive friend strengthens your bond. Pick a serene nature motif.

These personalized cards not only show that you value the recipient but also create cherished keepsakes.

Log Today's Activities and Experiences with The SPEAK Method

Use the questions or comments as a guide or write freely expressing your thoughts!

SELF-CARE – How did you act like a child today?

_____
_____
_____
_____
_____
_____
_____

PASSION – Who are the professionals you know who could give you an inspiring perspective?

_____
_____
_____
_____
_____
_____
_____
_____

EAT AND ENJOY NOURISHING FOOD – What are some of your favorite one pot meals? How will you make them healthy?

ACTIVITY – Which of the deep breathing exercises are you going to try first?

KINDNESS – List friends or family you are going to send a card.

_____
_____
_____
_____
_____
_____

ADDITIONAL NOTES

_____
_____
_____
_____
_____
_____

DAILY REPORT CARD OF LIFE – How did you SPEAK today?

Grade Your Day, no D's or F's Allowed!

- **A** – Amazing
- **B** – Better than yesterday
- **C** – Challenging but working on it

DAY 13

"What you do makes a difference, and you have to decide what kind of difference you want to make. Given the choice, I'd spend all my days working with animals for free."
Jane Goodall

SELF-CARE – PRACTICE IT DAILY

One of the simplest yet most luxurious ways to practice self-care is by taking a bath. A warm bath can provide physical relaxation, mental clarity, and emotional comfort, making it an ideal way to unwind and invest in your well-being.

Set the Mood:

- Create a calming atmosphere by dimming the lights and lighting some scented candles. Play soft music or nature sounds to enhance the soothing environment. This helps signal your brain that it's time to relax and let go of stress.

Choose the Right Ingredients:

- Add bath salts, essential oils, or bubble bath to the water. Epsom salts can relieve muscle tension, while essential oils like lavender or eucalyptus can promote relaxation and clear your mind. Although it's not typically considered a "guy thing," my husband takes a daily lavender bath.

Focus on Comfort:

- Ensure that the water temperature is just right for you—not too hot, not too cold. Consider adding a bath pillow for neck support and lay back comfortably. This will allow you to fully savor the experience without any discomfort.

Incorporate Mindfulness:

- Use this time to practice mindfulness or meditation. Focus on your breathing, feel the warmth of the water against your skin, and let your thoughts drift away. This can enhance the mental benefits of your bath, leaving you feeling refreshed and centered.

By dedicating some time to a well-prepared bath, you can transform an ordinary routine into a powerful self-care ritual that nurtures your body, mind, and spirit.

PASSION – DISCOVER AND IGNITE IT

If money were no object, the possibilities for how to spend your time become limitless, offering a world of exploration, creativity, and joy. When financial constraints are lifted, you can delve deeply into what truly ignites your passion and brings fulfillment.

Experiment with DIY projects:

- Take on do-it-yourself projects at home, such as crafting, cooking new recipes, or DIY home improvements. Experimenting with hands-on activities can help you discover talents and interests you didn't know you had.

Nature Exploration:

- Spending time in nature has numerous benefits for the mind and soul. Hiking, bird watching, gardening, or simply taking long walks can help clear your mind and rejuvenate your spirit. Nature often offers a sense of peace and inspiration that can lead to personal revelations and a deeper understanding of what you enjoy doing.

Volunteer Work:

- Engaging in volunteer activities can be incredibly rewarding and eye-opening. Whether it's working with children, animals, the elderly, or the environment, giving your time to help others can reveal what truly matters to you.

  While living in Southern California, I enjoyed volunteering at a Boys and Girls Club for an after-school activity, where my passion for healthy food was further reinforced. The activity involved creating enchanted broccoli forests entirely out of food. By the end, even the pickiest eaters were enjoying the "broccoli trees" and "dirt" made from brown rice!

Think about how you can create your own
"if money were no object" endeavors.

EAT AND ENJOY – NOURISHING FOOD

Starting your day with a nourishing breakfast is crucial for maintaining optimal health and energy levels throughout the day. Breakfast kick-starts your metabolism, provides essential nutrients, and helps sustain productivity. Skipping breakfast can lead to fatigue, poor performance, and cravings for unhealthy snacks later.

Overnight Oats:

- Prepare this the night before by mixing rolled oats with your choice of milk (dairy or plant-based) and adding fruits, nuts, and a drizzle of honey. In the morning, you'll have a ready-to-eat, nutrient-packed breakfast. I make a point to prepare two or three jars at a time.

Smoothie Bowl:

- Blend your favorite fruits with a base of yogurt or milk, then pour the smoothie into a bowl. Top it with granola, chia seeds, and fresh berries for added texture and nutritional benefits. It's a quick, tasty, and customizable option.

Make Ahead Breakfast Casseroles:

- Make-ahead casseroles are a fantastic way to ensure you have several days' worth of hearty breakfasts ready to go. These dishes can be prepared in advance and simply heated up in the morning, saving you valuable time during busy weekdays.
- Delicious options to consider: French toast casserole, baked oatmeal, breakfast burrito casserole and my family's favorite **Amish Breakfast Casserole.**

Greek Yogurt Parfait:

- Layer Greek yogurt with fresh fruits, nuts, and a bit of granola for crunch. Greek yogurt is high in protein and probiotics, making it an excellent choice for a quick, balanced breakfast.

Give these make-ahead quick ideas a try, and you'll find breakfast time becomes a breeze!

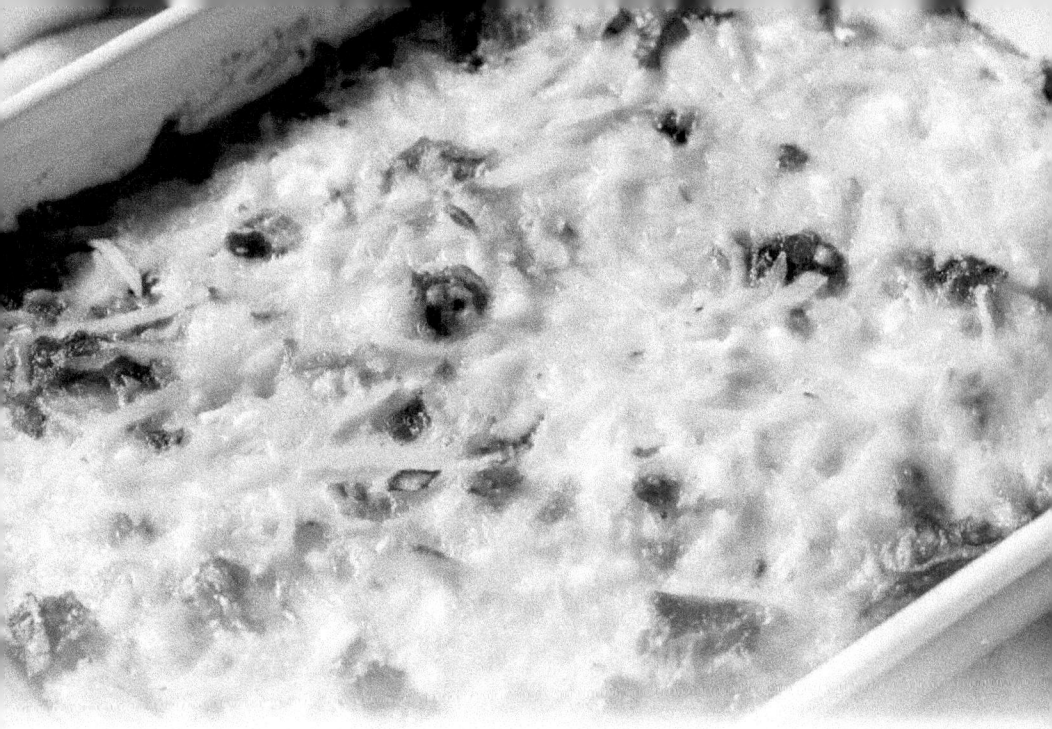

Amish Breakfast Casserole

8-10 Servings

INGREDIENTS:

- 6 large eggs
- 4 cups frozen shredded hash brown potatoes, thawed
- 3 cups shredded sharp cheddar cheese (can use 1 cup shredded Swiss and 2 cups shredded cheddar)
- 1-1/2 cups cottage cheese
- 1 bunch green onions, sliced thin including greens
- 1/2 teaspoon sea salt
- 1/4 teaspoon ground black pepper
- Optional: 6 slices sugar free bacon, cooked until crisp and crumbled
- Optional: 2 cups chopped fresh spinach

PROCESS:

1. Preheat oven to 350°F.
2. In a large bowl, beat eggs until foamy.

3. Add cheese and mix well.
4. Add onions, thawed potatoes, salt and pepper and mix just to incorporate and optional chopped spinach
5. Transfer to an oiled 13x9-in. baking dish.
6. Optional: top with crisp bacon crumbles.
7. Bake, uncovered in preheated oven until a knife inserted in the center comes out clean, 35-40 minutes.
8. Let stand for 10 minutes before cutting.

HINT: Casserole can be assembled the night before. Take out of the fridge for 30 minutes before baking in preheated oven.

ACTIVITY – EMBRACE AND LOVE MOVEMENT

Martial arts offer a dynamic way to stay active while developing both physical and mental skills. These practices combine elements of fitness, self-defense, discipline, and mindfulness, making them a well-rounded activity for individuals of all ages. Whether you're looking to enhance your physical fitness, learn self-defense, or find a new way to relieve stress, martial arts can be an excellent choice.

Watch You Tube videos to find one that resonates with you.

Karate:

- Focuses on striking techniques using punches, kicks, knees, and elbows. It's ideal for individuals seeking a disciplined approach to self-defense and those looking to improve their overall physical strength, coordination, and mental focus.

Taekwondo:

- Known for its high and fast kicks, this Korean martial art emphasizes agility and flexibility. It's perfect for individuals who prioritize speed, precision, and martial arts that incorporate acrobatic moves, making it popular among younger practitioners and athletes.

Brazilian Jiu-Jitsu

- A grappling-based art that focuses on ground fighting and submission holds. It's well-suited for those interested in gaining proficiency in close-combat techniques and leveraging one's body mechanics, making it a favorite among mixed martial artists and self-defense enthusiasts.

Kung Fu:

- Encompasses various Chinese martial arts styles, it's characterized by fluid movements and powerful strikes. It's great for individuals who appreciate a holistic approach to martial arts, integrating philosophy, agility, and strength, often appealing to those attracted to traditional martial arts culture.

Embarking on a martial arts journey can be incredibly rewarding, providing you with lifelong benefits both physically and mentally.

KINDNESS – CULTIVATE IT IN YOUR DAILY LIFE

Hosting a 'Free Yard Sale' is a wonderful act of kindness that not only allows you to declutter your home but also provides much needed items to those who could benefit from them. By giving away gently used possessions, you can make a significant impact in your community.

Gather and Prepare Items:

- Begin by sorting through your belongings and selecting items that are in good condition but no longer needed. This could include clothes, toys, kitchenware, books, and electronics. Make sure items are clean and in good condition.

Promote Your Event:

- Spread the word about your 'Free Yard Sale' through social media, local community boards, and word of mouth. Inform neighbors, friends, and local organizations that work with individuals in need. Clearly state the date, time, and location of your event.

Create an Inviting Setup:

- Arrange your items neatly and clearly label different sections to make it easy for visitors to browse. Consider setting up tables and providing bags for people to carry their selections. Play some uplifting music and decorate your yard to create a welcoming atmosphere.

Involve the Community:

- Encourage neighbors to participate by donating their unused items, volunteering to help with setup and clean-up, or simply promoting the event. This act of kindness can foster a greater sense of community and bring people together for a positive cause.

Hosting a 'Free Yard Sale' not only helps those in need but also brings your community closer and reinforces the spirit of generosity and sharing.

Log Today's Activities and Experiences with The SPEAK Method

Use the questions or comments as a guide or write freely expressing your thoughts!

SELF-CARE - Schedule your bath. List the items to make your bath a special self-care ritual.

_____
_____
_____
_____
_____
_____
_____

PASSION - List your *"if money were no object"* endeavors.

_____
_____
_____
_____
_____
_____
_____
_____

EAT AND ENJOY NOURISHING FOOD - What are your favorite breakfast foods? Are they healthy?

_____
_____
_____
_____
_____
_____
_____
_____

ACTIVITY – What simple martial arts moves are you going to try?

_____
_____
_____
_____
_____
_____
_____
_____

KINDNESS – What neighbors are you going to talk to about free yard sale?

_____
_____
_____
_____
_____
_____

ADDITIONAL NOTES

_____
_____
_____
_____
_____
_____

DAILY REPORT CARD OF LIFE – How did you SPEAK today?

Grade Your Day, no D's or F's Allowed!

- **A** – Amazing
- **B** – Better than yesterday
- **C** – Challenging but working on it

DAY 14

"Life is what happens when you're busy making other plans."
John Lennon

SELF-CARE – PRACTICE IT DAILY

Taking a day trip is an energizing self-care practice that provides a welcome break from routine and an opportunity to recharge. Moreover, day trips stimulate creativity and inspiration. By experiencing new sights, sounds, and environments, you can ignite your imagination and bring fresh ideas back into your daily life.

Nature Hike:

- Spend the day at a nearby state or national park. Stop by the visitor center for info. Hiking in fresh air, surrounded by nature, offers a chance to disconnect from technology and reconnect with yourself and the environment.

Beach or Lake Day:

- Being near the beach or a lake can be incredibly rejuvenating. The sound of the waves, the feeling of sand under your feet, and the fresh air create a relaxing experience. Bring a book, a picnic, and plenty of sunscreen.

Cultural Exploration:

- Visit a nearby city or town you haven't explored before. Spend the day visiting museums, art galleries, and historical sites. Engaging with new cultural experiences can stimulate your mind while providing physical activity. Living near Asheville, North Carolina, offers me abundant cultural exploration opportunities, including the Biltmore, the largest privately owned house in the US, and the 101-year-old Grove Park Inn. Look for ones near you.

Wellness Retreat:

- Look for a local spa or wellness center offering day-long retreats. Activities might include yoga, meditation, massages, or other therapeutic treatments. Invest a day in pampering yourself.

Each of these day trips provide an excellent opportunity to break free from your usual routine.

PASSION – DISCOVER AND IGNITE IT

Creating a personal mission statement, no matter your stage in life, is a powerful way to define your passion and direct your life's purpose. It serves as a compass, aligning your values with your actions and helping you stay focused on what truly matters.

Reflect on Your Values:

- Start by identifying what is most important to you. Consider your core beliefs, principles, and the values that drive your daily actions. For instance, you might value integrity, compassion, and continuous learning.

Identify Your Strengths and Passions:

- Take inventory of your skills, talents, and passions. What activities make you lose track of time? What do you excel at naturally? Understanding what you are good at and what you love to do will provide a strong foundation for your mission statement.

Keep it Concise:

- Combine your values, strengths, and vision into a concise statement. It should be clear, specific, and inspirational. Keep it short and powerful, typically one to two sentences. Aim to capture the essence of what drives you. I keep fine tuning mine, "To leverage my passion for cooking, alongside my expertise in healthy living, to inspire and transform lives."

Write and Refine Your Statement:

- Crafting your own mission statement involves introspection and clarity. Don't worry about getting it perfect on the first try; it's a process of refinement until it genuinely reflects your passions and motivates you to reach your goals.

By following these steps you'll craft a personal mission statement that captures the essence of your passions.

EAT AND ENJOY – NOURISHING FOOD

Switching to a plant-based diet one day a week can be a powerful way to improve your health, protect the environment, and explore new culinary adventures. This simple commitment can bring a variety of benefits without feeling overwhelming, encouraging a more mindful approach to eating.

Focus on Whole Foods:

- Base your meals around whole foods such as fruits, vegetables, legumes, nuts, seeds, and whole grains. These foods are nutritious, filling, and versatile. Avoid overly processed plant-based options, which can be high in sugars and unhealthy fats.

Swap Out Dairy and Meat Alternatives:

- Try using almond milk, oat milk, or soy milk instead of dairy milk. Experiment with tofu, tempeh, seitan, or legumes like chickpeas and lentils as replacements for meat in your favorite dishes. These alternatives can provide the necessary protein and flavor.

Go International:

- Use this opportunity to get creative in the kitchen. Explore cuisines known for their plant-based dishes, such as Mediterranean, Indian, or Thai. Incorporating diverse flavors can make your plant-based day exciting and enjoyable.

Combine Proteins:

- When eating plant-based, it's important to combine different protein sources to get a complete protein profile. You can try chickpea or lentil pasta topped with marinara sauce and pine nuts. My personal favorite is **Black Bean and Quinoa Burgers.** My family does not even miss the meat!

Starting with just one day a week can make a big difference over time.

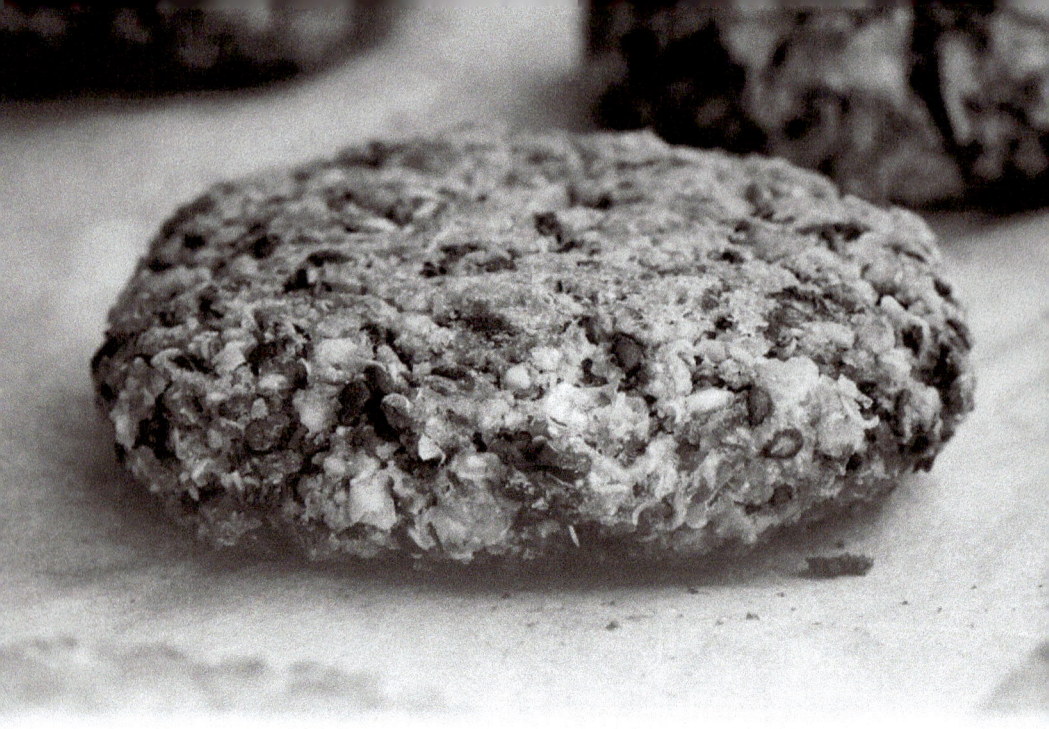

Salsa Black Bean Burgers

8 Servings

INGREDIENTS:

- ½ cup prepared salsa
- 2 (15 ounce) cans black beans, drained and rinsed
- 1 cup well-crushed tortilla chips
- ½ cup grated white onion
- 1 large egg, beaten
- 3 Tablespoons sugar free mayonnaise
- 4 teaspoons chili powder
- 2 teaspoons ground cumin
- ¾ teaspoon salt
- 3 Tablespoons avocado oil, divided
- 8 whole-grain burger buns, wraps or English muffins, toasted
- ½ cup prepared guacamole
- 8 slices tomato slices
- 1 cup sprouts
- ½ cup thinly sliced red onion

PROCESS:

1. Place salsa in a fine-mesh sieve and stir a few times to drain excess liquid.
2. Mash beans with a potato masher in a large bowl until no whole ones remain.
3. Stir in the drained salsa, crushed tortilla chips, grated onion, egg, mayonnaise, chili powder, cumin and salt. Let stand 10 minutes.
4. Form the bean mixture into 8 burgers about 3 inches wide (⅓ cup each).
5. Heat 1½ Tablespoons oil in a large nonstick skillet over medium-high heat.
6. Reduce heat to medium, add 4 burgers and cook until browned and heated through, 3 to 4 minutes per side.
7. Repeat with the remaining oil and burgers.
8. Serve the burgers on buns, wraps or muffins with guacamole, tomato slices, sprouts and red onion.
9. To make ahead: Individually wrap cooked burgers and refrigerate for up to 5 days or freeze for up to 3 months.
10. Microwave or bake to reheat.

ACTIVITY – EMBRACE AND LOVE MOVEMENT

Geocaching is an engaging outdoor adventure game that blends technology with exploration, making it a fantastic way to stay active and discover new places in your area. The game involves searching for hidden treasures, called "geocaches," using GPS-enabled devices. With millions of geocaches hidden worldwide, this modern-day treasure hunt provides endless opportunities for excitement, exercise, and adventure. I discovered that there are over 1300 geocaches in my area.

Download a Geocaching App:

- Download a geocaching app like Geocaching® or Cachly. Create a free account to access the full range of geocaching features. These apps provide maps, coordinates, and clues to help you find hidden geocaches near you.

Check the Difficulty and Terrain Ratings:

- Geocaches are rated based on their difficulty and the terrain you'll encounter. Start with easier and more accessible caches to familiarize yourself with the process.

Bring a Pen and Small Trade Items:

- Many geocaches contain a logbook to sign, so always carry a pen. Additionally, some caches have small trade items. If you take something, be sure to leave something of equal or greater value for the next geocacher.

Dress the Part:

- Choose sturdy, comfortable shoes or hiking boots that provide good traction and support. Wear durable, flexible pants or shorts that allow for easy movement. Protect yourself from the sun by wearing a wide-brimmed hat, sunglasses, and sunscreen.

Whether you're a solo explorer or enjoy activities with friends and family, geocaching offers a unique and fun way to get moving and engage with your surroundings.

KINDNESS – CULTIVATE IT IN YOUR DAILY LIFE

Regularly donating blood or plasma is a life-saving act of kindness that can make a significant difference for those in need, especially during times of critical shortage. Every donation can help save lives, support medical treatments, and improve the health outcomes of patients in hospitals. By becoming a regular donor, you contribute to a reliable and sustainable supply of blood and plasma.

Find a Reputable Donation Center:

- Locate a certified blood or plasma donation center in your area. Well-known organizations like the Red Cross, hospitals, and specialized plasma centers are excellent options to ensure your donation is safe and beneficial. Most centers have a donation age requirement of 18-65.

Schedule an Appointment:

- By scheduling an appointment, you streamline the donation process and reduce wait times. Many donation centers allow you to book your appointment online, making it convenient to find a suitable time.

Prepare for Your Donation:

- Ensure you are hydrated, have eaten a healthy meal, and are well-rested before your donation. Avoid heavy physical activity and alcohol consumption the day before. Bringing a valid ID and understanding the health requirements are also essential.

Post-Donation Care:

- After donating, relax and take advantage of the refreshments provided. Hydrate well and avoid strenuous activities for the rest of the day. Following these guidelines helps ensure a positive donation experience and quick recovery.

By following these steps, you can make a regular commitment to donating blood or plasma, saving lives, and supporting your community in times of need.

Log Today's Activities and Experiences with The SPEAK Method

Use the questions or comments as a guide or write freely expressing your thoughts!

SELF-CARE – Where are you going on your day trips?

PASSION – Write the first draft of your mission statement.

EAT AND ENJOY NOURISHING FOOD
List your plant-based meal favorites.

ACTIVITY – What Geocaches app did you download? When do you plan and getting your "caches"?

KINDNESS – When are you going to donate plasma or blood.

ADDITIONAL NOTES

DAILY REPORT CARD OF LIFE – How did you SPEAK today?

Grade Your Day, no D's or F's Allowed!

- **A** – Amazing
- **B** – Better than yesterday
- **C** – Challenging but working on it

Interview
Dr. Katelyn – Doctor of Chiropractic, Bachelors of Behavioral Neuroscience.

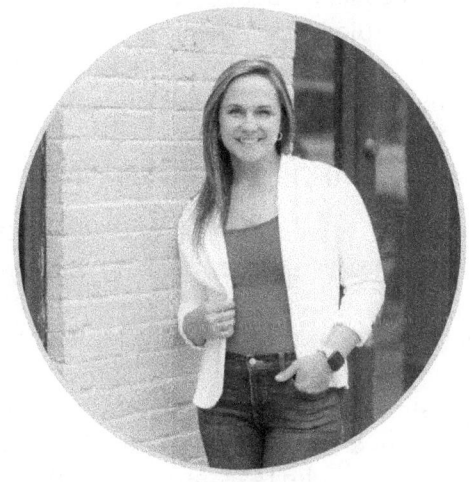

SELF-CARE – PRACTICE IT DAILY

I get regular massages, exercise and have physical therapy with dry needling to help maintain my body due to having a job where I need to use it all the time. It is also important for me to get 7-8 hours' sleep a night and suggest the same to my patients. Drinking enough water and replacing electrolytes are basics that I also follow and teach to my patients

PASSION – DISCOVER AND IGNITE IT

I always knew I wanted to help people. When I became a fitness coach after undergraduate school, I discovered how the body heals itself when we take care of it. Through my own injuries and learning to heal them with chiropractic care, massage and exercise, this belief was solidified. Teaching people how to heal themselves remains a vital part of my passion and practice.

Bowling is another of my passions. I have been bowling since I was 5 and continued through college in Iowa on a bowling scholarship at St. Ambrose University. Now, I continue to bowl in a local league and recently achieved my first perfect 300 score! I attribute this success not just to practice but to truly enjoying life to its fullest.

EAT AND ENJOY - NOURISHING FOOD

I engage in simple meal prep, focusing on preparing proteins. I also make it a point to limit sugar and alcohol intake. I adhere to and teach the 80/20 rule: 80% consume lean proteins and whole foods, and 20% enjoy foods of my choice. Allowing occasional splurges makes the approach more sustainable.

ACTIVITY – EMBRACE AND LOVE MOVEMENT

I stress to patients the importance of movement, even 5-10 minutes a day of stretching/ resistance training can make a world of difference and prevent issues down the road. I am also a big advocate for resistance training. Many times, people are resistant to do resistance training as they don't want to "bulk up." Training once a week to build stronger muscles is enough to help your body have stronger joints and stronger bones due to having to maintain the strength you achieve with resistance training. Leading to more longevity and being able to enjoy life as you age. It can also help your muscles store vital nutrients to help you when your levels get depleted.

KINDNESS – CULTIVATE IT IN YOUR DAILY LIFE

Toxic relationships are just like any other stress on the body and can cause an increase in cortisol. You need to get rid of them and form fun, loving relationships. Unfortunately, we are at a time in history where people are experiencing more loneliness than we ever have before. We were locked inside, forced to not be around other people and we wore masks and could not see smiles for too long. A smile and a conversation can go a long way to improve your overall health. It is important to keep connected so I make it a point to plan dinner with girlfriends at least once a month. Something as simple as giving compliments spreads kindness.

www.dynamicchirofm.com

dynamicchirofm@gmail.com

DAY 15

"Solitude is where I place my chaos to rest and awaken my inner peace."
Edna O'Brien

SELF-CARE – PRACTICE IT DAILY

Taking time for solitude is a crucial aspect of self-care that allows for deep reflection, mental clarity, and emotional well-being. Amidst the constant demands of daily life, carving out moments for oneself can rejuvenate the mind and spirit, fostering a sense of inner peace and balance.

Morning Meditations:

- Start your day with a few minutes of meditation in a quiet space. Sit comfortably, close your eyes, and focus on your breath. This practice helps clear your mind, setting a calm and focused tone for the rest of the day.

Nature Walks:

- Spend time in nature by going for a walk in a nearby park or nature reserve. Being in nature allows you to reconnect with yourself. Make sure to choose a safe environment and carry personal identification.

Dedicated Reading Time:

- Create a designated reading nook in your home where you can retreat with a good book. Reading not only offers the joy of escaping into another world but also provides a quiet space where you can be alone with your thoughts.

Solo Creative Activities:

- Engage in activities like painting, knitting, or journaling. These creative outlets allow you to express yourself freely and reflectively without external distractions. I personally love being in the kitchen alone, creating new recipes. However, I do allow my dog Mollie to watch in case I drop a crumb.

By integrating these moments of solitude into your routine, you'll find yourself more grounded, centered, and equipped to handle the responsibilities of everyday life.

PASSION – DISCOVER AND IGNITE IT

Finding your true passion can be a rewarding journey, and seeking advice from those around you can provide valuable insights and perspectives. Friends, family, and co-workers often see our strengths and interests from different angles, making their input essential in uncovering what truly excites you.

Be Specific:

- When seeking advice, be clear about what you're looking for. Instead of broadly asking for career advice, narrow it down to specific areas of interest. For example, "I'm exploring my interest in cooking and nutrition, do you think this aligns with my strengths?"

Set Up a Comfortable Environment:

- Create a relaxed and open atmosphere for the conversation. Whether it's over a casual coffee or a quiet lunch, a comfortable setting encourages honest and thoughtful exchanges.

Ask Open-Ended Questions:

- Frame your questions to elicit detailed responses. Questions like, "What activities have you noticed I lose track of time doing?" or "When have you seen me the happiest or most engaged?" can lead to deeper insights into your passions.

Remain Open and Non-Defensive:

- Approach these discussions with an open mind. Be prepared for feedback that may not align with your current views and avoid getting attached to a specific outcome or feeling offended. Use their input as a tool for reflection rather than absolute guidance.

By engaging with those who know you well, you'll gain a broader perspective on your interests and talents, paving the way to discovering your true passion.

EAT AND ENJOY – NOURISHING FOOD

Eating out can be a delightful experience, but it often poses challenges when aiming to make healthy choices. When I owned my restaurant, Season's Best, in a lively university town, I quickly learned the importance of being flexible and accommodating to customers' healthy requests.

Fresh Ingredients:

- Explore restaurants that prioritize fresh, seasonal ingredients. Menus featuring farm-to-table or locally sourced items usually indicate that the food will be nutritious and flavorful. Choose gluten-free or vegetarian meals and substitute vegetables for the loaded baked potato.

Choose Healthy Cooking Methods:

- Avoid fried and breaded items or dishes drowning in creamy, sugary, or oily sauces.

  Look for cooking methods that involve grilling, baking, or steaming.

Oversized Portions:

- Consider sharing a dish or requesting a half portion. Another option is to ask for a takeout box when you order your meal and place half of it in the box before you start eating, allowing you to enjoy the rest later.

Sugary Drinks and Desserts:

- Skip sugary beverages and calorie-laden desserts. Choose water, unsweetened tea, or sparkling water and consider fresh fruit or a smaller, lighter dessert option.

Make it at Home:

- If you're not in the mood to dine out, try recreating a favorite restaurant dish at home, such as a twist on the famous pasta chain soup, **Cauliflower Zuppa Toscana.**

Follow these healthier choices while enjoying the pleasure of dining out.

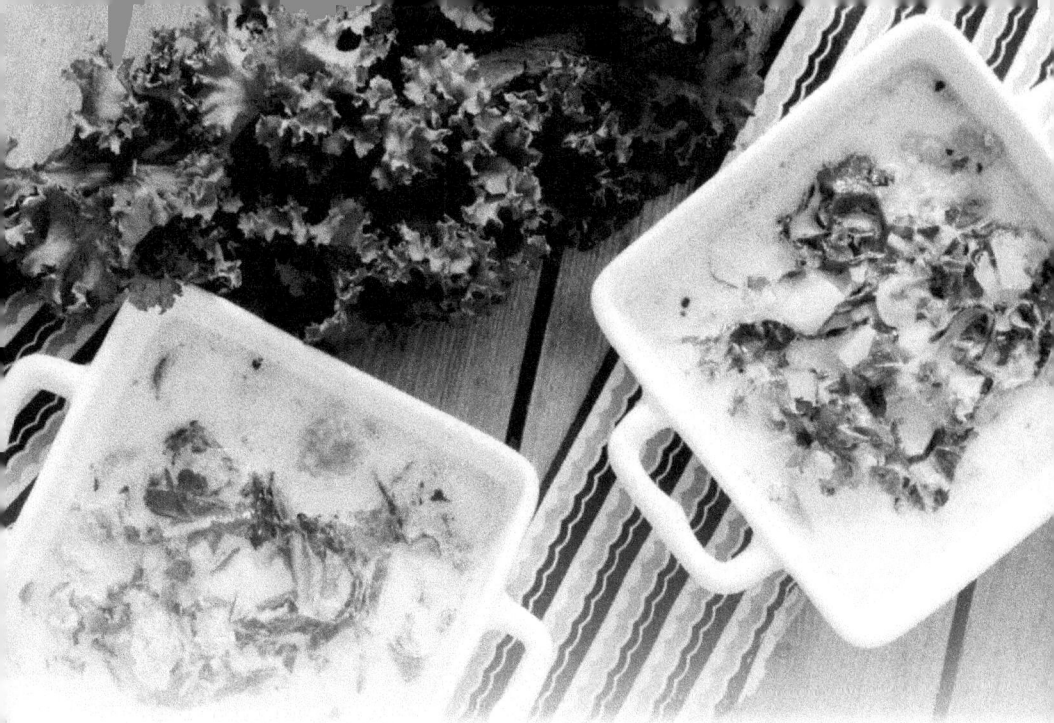

Cauliflower Zuppa Toscana Soup

6 Servings

INGREDIENTS:

- 1 pound chicken or turkey sausage (or use ground chicken or turkey)
- 1 Tablespoon olive oil
- ½ cup onion, finely diced
- 3 garlic cloves, minced
- 4 cups chicken broth
- 1 large cauliflower head, diced into small florets
- 3 cups chopped kale
- ¼ teaspoon crushed red pepper flakes
- 1 Tablespoon Italian Seasoning
- 1 teaspoon thyme leaf ½ to
- 1 teaspoon salt to taste ¼ teaspoon pepper
- 1 cup ½ and ½
- ¼ cup chopped fresh parsley

PROCESS:

1. Brown the sausage in a stock pot over medium heat until done.

2. Remove from pan and drain sausage.
3. Heat olive oil in same pan and sauté onions and garlic until onions are barely translucent.
4. Scrape up any bits of sausage. Add broth, cauliflower florets, spices, salt and pepper and stir to combine.
5. Cook on medium heat for 15-20 minutes until cauliflower is fork tender.
6. Turn heat to low and add kale, cooked sausage and ½ and ½.
7. Cook just long enough to wilt kale. DO NOT BOIL. Serve garnished with fresh parsley.

ACTIVITY – EMBRACE AND LOVE MOVEMENT

Chair exercises are an excellent way to stay active, especially if you have joint issues or feel exhausted at the end of the day. Low-impact movements can help improve flexibility, strength, and circulation without putting added strain on your body. Explore YouTube videos for targeted exercises or consider trying a free month of the BetterMe app.

Chair Yoga:

- Try seated forward bends to stretch your back and hamstrings, or gentle chair twists to release tension in your spine. Breathing exercises performed while seated can also help you relax and reduce stress.

Chair Pilates:

- Begin with seated marches, lifting each knee, one at a time, toward your chest. Another exercise involves lifting your right leg and touching your toes with your left hand, then alternating sides.

Seated Arm and Leg Extensions:

- Target your core without straining your knees. Sit straight in your chair and extend your arms parallel to your shoulders. While keeping your arms extended, slowly extend your legs out in front of you with knees slightly bent. To the count of five, lower both your arms and legs, then, again to the count of five, slowly raise them back to the starting position.

Arm Circles:

- Sit upright and stretch your arms out to the sides. Make small circular motions with your arms, gradually increasing the size of the circles. Reverse the direction after a few seconds.

Incorporating chair exercises into your routine will help you stay active, alleviate joint pain, and rejuvenate your body after a long day.

KINDNESS – CULTIVATE IT IN YOUR DAILY LIFE

One simple and impactful way to spread kindness and joy is by purchasing a $10 gift card each month and leaving it on a store shelf with a heartfelt note. Sacrificing just one fast food meal or coffee shop latte can make this small gesture possible and brighten someone's day, creating a ripple effect of kindness and positivity in your community. Each $10 gift card you leave behind is more than just a monetary gift; it is a symbol of hope and generosity that can transform someone's day.

Vary the Locations:

- Choose different stores each month; a grocery store, a bookstore, a pharmacy, or a café, ensuring more people have the chance to experience an unexpected moment of joy.

Personalize Your Note:

- Write a warm and encouraging message to accompany the gift card. Mention how you hope it helps the recipient and wish them a wonderful day. Personal touches can make the gesture even more meaningful.

Choose Busy Times:

- Place the gift card on the shelf during peak shopping hours. This increases the likelihood that someone will find it quickly and have their day brightened without much delay.

Be Discreet:

- Quietly place the gift card on a shelf without drawing attention to yourself. This ensures the act remains anonymous and feels like a genuine surprise for the person who finds it.

This thoughtful act can inspire others to pay it forward, spreading happiness and generosity far beyond what you might expect.

Log Today's Activities and Experiences with The SPEAK Method

Use the questions or comments as a guide or write freely expressing your thoughts!

SELF-CARE – How many minutes of solitude are you going to take and where?

_____
_____
_____
_____
_____
_____
_____

PASSION – List friends and family you feel comfortable asking for advice.

_____
_____
_____
_____
_____
_____
_____
_____

EAT AND ENJOY NOURISHING FOOD – What are your favorite restaurant meals and how will you make the best choices when eating out?

ACTIVITY – List exercise you will do in a chair.

KINDNESS – Where are you going to leave your first anonymous gift card?

ADDITIONAL NOTES

DAILY REPORT CARD OF LIFE – How did you SPEAK today?

Grade Your Day, no D's or F's Allowed!

- **A** – Amazing
- **B** – Better than yesterday
- **C** – Challenging but working on it

DAY 16

> "The mind is not a vessel to be filled,
> but a fire to be kindled."
> **Plato**

SELF-CARE – PRACTICE IT DAILY

Taking care of your mind is as crucial as maintaining physical health. A well-cared-for mind boosts creativity, enhances mood, and improves overall well-being. Engaging in mental self-care practices helps you manage stress, build resilience, and maintain focus.

Stay Hydrated:

- Since your brain is almost 80% water, drinking enough water is fundamental for brain health. Dehydration can lead to poor concentration, headaches, and mood swings. Carry a water bottle with you to ensure consistent hydration throughout the day.

Play Games:

- Engaging in mentally stimulating games like puzzles, chess, or word games can sharpen cognitive abilities and delay the onset of cognitive decline. These activities challenge your mind, improve problem-solving skills, and provide a fun and relaxing break from daily stressors. During my childhood, we frequently completed jigsaw puzzles, and my younger sister, Anne, became a true puzzle aficionado!

Practice Mindfulness:

- Mindfulness techniques like meditation and deep-breathing exercises help reduce stress and anxiety. By focusing on the present moment, you can foster a sense of calm and clarity. Incorporate a few minutes of mindfulness into your daily routine to enhance your mental resilience.

Get Adequate Sleep:

- Quality sleep is essential for mental recovery and cognitive function. Ensure you get 7-9 hours of sleep each night to improve memory, mood, and overall mental health. Create a consistent sleep schedule and a restful environment to enhance sleep quality. Remember to turn off all technology at least an hour before bed.

By integrating these self-care practices, you'll create a nurturing environment for your mind to thrive.

PASSION – DISCOVER AND IGNITE IT

Unlocking your passion begins with a deep understanding of your core values. These fundamental beliefs guide your behaviors, decisions, and priorities, acting as a compass to what truly matters in your life. By aligning your actions with your core values, you will unveil and fuel your passions.

Authenticity:

- **Sample Core Value: Integrity** - When you practice integrity, you remain true to who you are and what you believe in, without conforming to others' expectations. Ensure you are clear on your principles and consistently align your actions with them.

Curiosity:

- **Sample Core Value: Lifelong Learning** - The desire to learn and explore new horizons often points toward hidden passions. When I started my job as a health coach, I had no idea I would need to learn to manage multiple online systems. It turns out, I loved the challenge. You're never too old to learn!

Contribution:

- **Sample Core Value: Service** - Feeling a sense of purpose and making a meaningful impact can illuminate your passions. Think about the causes or communities you care about deeply. Look for volunteer opportunities that align with your passion.

Creativity:

- **Sample Core Value: Innovation** - Creative expression allows you to explore new ideas and perspectives, building a deeper connection with your passions. Whether it's through art, writing, or problem-solving, creativity opens doors to things you love.

By leveraging your core values, you can navigate the path to discovering what sets your soul on fire, ultimately leading a more passionate and fulfilling life.

EAT AND ENJOY – NOURISHING FOOD

Elevate your culinary experience by incorporating healthy sauces into your meals. These nutrient-rich additions enhance the flavor of your dishes and provide numerous health benefits. By choosing wholesome ingredients, you can enjoy a tasty and nutritious dining experience without compromising your health goals. Get ready to transform your meals.

Pesto:

- Made with fresh basil, garlic, pine nuts, olive oil, and Parmesan cheese, pesto is rich in healthy fats and adds a burst of flavor to pasta, vegetables, and proteins. Be creative with ingredients by trying additions like arugula, fresh spinach, or a variety of nuts.

Barbeque Sauce:

- This sauce adds tang and spice to meat and seafood. Different regions across the country have their own versions of BBQ sauce, whether tomato-based, vinegar, or honey mustard. However, many of these varieties contain high sugar content. For a healthier alternative, try my popular **Honey-Based Barbeque Sauce.**

Yogurt-Based Tzatziki:

- This Greek sauce made from plain yogurt, cucumber, garlic, and dill is high in protein and probiotics. It's a refreshing and nutritious addition to grilled meats, wraps, or as a dip for vegetables, offering a cool and creamy texture.

Coconut Curry Sauce:

- A simple sauce made from coconut milk, curry paste, garlic, and ginger provide a creamy, flavorful addition to stir-fries, vegetables, and seafood dishes while offering healthy fats. Additionally, the spices in this sauce have anti-inflammatory benefits.

Avoid boredom and sauce up your meals!

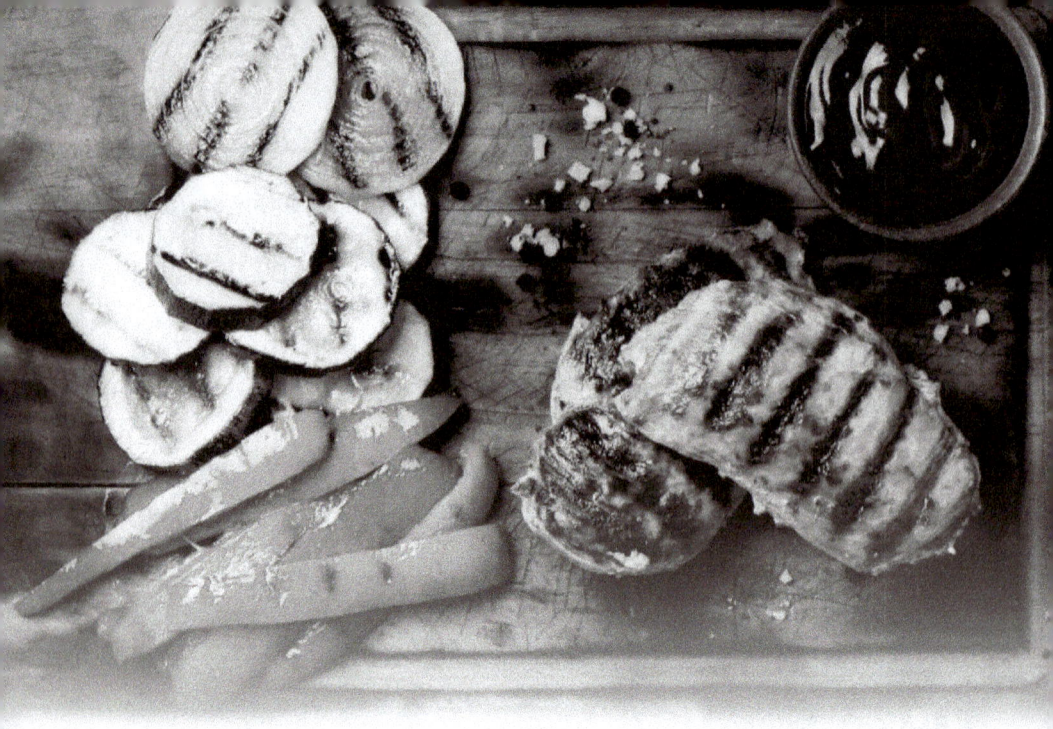

Honey Barbeque Sauce

Makes 2 Cups

INGREDIENTS:

- 1 Tablespoon coconut oil
- 1 cup yellow onion, finely chopped
- 3-4 cloves fresh garlic, minced
- 1 Tablespoon soy sauce or Tamari
- 1 teaspoon cumin
- 1 teaspoon oregano
- 1 teaspoon basil
- 1 teaspoon smoked paprika
- 1 teaspoon chipotle chili powder
- 1 Tablespoon chili powder
- ½ teaspoon celery salt
- 1 6 oz can tomato paste
- 1 ½ cup chicken or veggie stock
- 2 Tablespoons apple cider vinegar
- 2 Tablespoons honey

PROCESS:

1. Heat oil in saucepan and sauté onion 3-4 minutes until translucent, add garlic and sauté until lightly brown.
2. Add all remaining ingredients and bring to a slow boil.
3. You can serve like this but if you want a thicker sauce, cover and simmer on low heat for approximately 15 minutes. This melds the flavors for a thicker and delicious sauce.
4. If you want a less spicy sauce cut back on both chili powders. This sauce keeps in the fridge for about 2 weeks.

Use: 1-2 Tablespoons on one serving of the following:

- Mix with pulled rotisserie chicken for a quick chicken sandwich
- Brush on chicken breast or chicken tenders before and after grilling.

ACTIVITY – EMBRACE AND LOVE MOVEMENT

Volunteering at events or organizations that require physical work is an excellent way to incorporate movement into your day while making a meaningful impact on your community. You get the chance to stay active, connect with like-minded individuals and contribute to a greater cause.

Community Clean-Up Events:

- Participating in local clean-up initiatives helps beautify your neighborhood and protect the environment. Activities often include picking up litter, planting trees, or maintaining community gardens. These tasks require a bit of physical effort, making it a perfect way to get your daily exercise.

Charity Runs and Walks:

- Many non-profits organize runs and walks to raise funds and awareness for their causes. Volunteering at these events can involve various physical tasks, such as setting up stations, handing out water to participants, or even joining the run or walk yourself.

Building and Repair Projects:

- Organizations like Habitat for Humanity often require volunteers for construction or repair projects. Whether you're building homes, painting walls, or performing minor repairs, these activities offer a full-body workout and the satisfaction of seeing your hard work materialize.

Food Banks and Meal Programs:

- Volunteering at food banks or meal programs often involves lifting and moving food supplies, packing boxes, or serving meals. The physical activities associated with these tasks not only help keep you moving but also provide vital support to those in need.

By choosing volunteer opportunities that require physical work, you can seamlessly integrate movement into your day while positively impacting those around you.

KINDNESS – CULTIVATE IT IN YOUR DAILY LIFE

Social media has become a primary means of communication for many, allowing individuals to share their thoughts, views, and experiences with a wide audience. While it offers an incredible platform for connection, it can sometimes foster negativity. By focusing on kindness, we can help create a more supportive and positive online environment.

Think Before You Post:

- Before sharing anything, consider the impact your words or images might have on others. Ask yourself if your post is helpful, encouraging, or supportive. Avoid sharing content that could be harmful or offensive.

Engage Positively:

- Like, share, and comment on posts that uplift and inspire. Compliment others on their achievements, offer words of encouragement, and show genuine interest in what they have to say. Your positive engagement can uplift someone's day. I always look forward to my friend Vicki's daily posts filled with inspiring quotes or affirmations and make sure to like them.

Promote Constructive Discussions:

- When engaging in conversations that involve differing opinions, maintain respect and an open mind. Be willing to listen and understand others' perspectives. Use polite language, avoid personal attacks, and stay calm even when disagreements arise.

Report and Block Negativity:

- Protecting your mental well-being is just as important as spreading kindness. If you encounter harmful or abusive behavior, report it to the platform's moderators and consider blocking the user. This not only safeguards your peace but also helps maintain a respectful community for others.

By committing to these practices, we can contribute to a kinder and more inclusive social media landscape.

Log Today's Activities and Experiences with The SPEAK Method

Use the questions or comments as a guide or write freely expressing your thoughts!

SELF-CARE – What puzzles or mind games do you enjoy?

_____
_____
_____
_____
_____
_____
_____

PASSION – List your core values.

_____
_____
_____
_____
_____
_____
_____
_____

EAT AND ENJOY NOURISHING FOOD – List your favorite sauces. Check their sugar content.

_____

_____

_____

_____

_____

_____

_____

_____

_____

ACTIVITY – What volunteer events are in your area?

_____

_____

_____

_____

_____

_____

_____

_____

_____

KINDNESS – CULTIVATE IT IN YOUR DAILY LIFE – How were you kind on social media?

_____
_____
_____
_____
_____

ADDITIONAL NOTES

_____
_____
_____
_____
_____
_____

DAILY REPORT CARD OF LIFE – How did you SPEAK today?

Grade Your Day, no D's or F's Allowed!

    A – Amazing
    B – Better than yesterday
    C – Challenging but working on it

DAY 17

"Without patience, we will learn less in life. We will see less. We will feel less. We will hear less."
Mother Teresa

SELF-CARE – PRACTICE IT DAILY

Taking a nap is an excellent self-care activity that helps rejuvenate your mind and body. Even if you don't fully fall asleep, the act of resting can be immensely beneficial. As you might notice, I love acronyms. My acronym for a NAP is: "Now at Peace." Even if you don't completely fall asleep, simply relaxing with your eyes closed is peaceful and enhances your productivity and stress levels.

Set a Proper Environment:

- Create a peaceful napping space by eliminating distractions, dimming lights, and setting a comfortable ambient temperature. This environment helps you relax and maximize the rejuvenating effects of a nap.

Keep it Short:

- Aiming for a nap duration of approximately 20-30 minutes ensures you don't fall into a deep sleep cycle, which can lead to grogginess upon waking. A short nap refreshes you without the potential of disrupting your nighttime sleep.

Listen to Your Body:

- Nap whenever your body signals the need for rest, such as when you feel drowsy in the early afternoon. This natural dip in alertness is part of your circadian rhythm, making it an optimal time for resting and recharging.

Gentle Awakening:

- Set a soothing alarm to ensure you wake up gently and peacefully. Use calming sounds or soft music rather than jarring alarms, allowing you to transition smoothly from rest to wakefulness and carry that peaceful state into the rest of your day.

Incorporating naps into your routine can significantly boost your mental and physical health, providing a welcoming respite in your busy schedule.

PASSION – DISCOVER AND IGNITE IT

Discovering your passion is a deeply personal and often transformative journey. It's crucial to be patient and understand that this process isn't about reaching the destination but embracing the journey itself. By prioritizing progress over perfection, you cultivate a more fulfilling exploration of your true interests.

Embrace Uncertainty:

- Understand that it's okay not to have all the answers right away. Uncertainty is a natural part of the discovery process. If you allow it, being comfortable with the unknown will open new and unexpected paths.

Set Small Goals:

- Break your journey into manageable steps by setting small, achievable goals. This approach reduces overwhelm and provides a clear roadmap. Accomplishing these mini goals can keep you motivated and focused.

Be Kind to Yourself:

- Recognize that finding your passion is a journey marked by trial and error. Allow yourself to make mistakes and learn from them. Celebrate small victories along the way and maintain a positive attitude even when faced with setbacks.

Take a Walk:

- One of my favorite sayings by Hippocrates is, "If you are in a bad mood, go for a walk. If you are still in a bad mood, go for another walk." While writing this book, I adapted his quote to say, "If you are impatient, go for a walk. If you are still impatient, go for another walk." Whenever I felt impatient about my writing progress, I took a walk. It's amazing how even a 10-minute walk can refresh and clear your mind.

EAT AND ENJOY – NOURISHING FOOD

Eating seasonal foods is a delightful and healthy way to reconnect with nature's cycle and enjoy produce at its peak freshness. Seasonal eating not only enhances the flavor and nutrition of your meals but also supports local farmers.

Winter:
- Root Vegetables: Carrots, beets, turnips and parsnips are perfect for roasting or stews.
- Citrus Fruits: Oranges, grapefruits, and lemons provide a burst of vitamin C. Juice or enjoy fresh.
- Dark Leafy Greens: Kale, collards, and Swiss chard offer a wealth of nutrients and can be used in soups, sautés, or salads.

Spring:
- Asparagus: Full of fiber, asparagus is great steamed, grilled or roasted.
- Strawberries: Rich in antioxidants and can be enjoyed fresh, in smoothies, or desserts.
- Peas: Fresh peas add a sweet, crisp texture to stir-fries and salads.

Summer
- Tomatoes: Nothing says summer more than a tomato. Great for salads, sauces, and BLT's. A favorite memory is my niece Michelle and me going out to the garden with a saltshaker and eating tomatoes straight off the vine. Try a cooking class favorite, **Tuscan Tomato Bread Salad.**
- Berries: Blueberries, raspberries, and blackberries are low in sugar and perfect for snacking, baking, or adding to yogurt.

Fall:
- Pumpkins: High in vitamin A; ideal for soups, pies, and roasting.
- Apples: Great for eating fresh, baking or making applesauce.
- Squash: Butternut, acorn, and spaghetti squash varieties offer hearty options for roasting or mashing.

Embrace the flavors of each season and enjoy the benefits of eating what nature provides at its best.

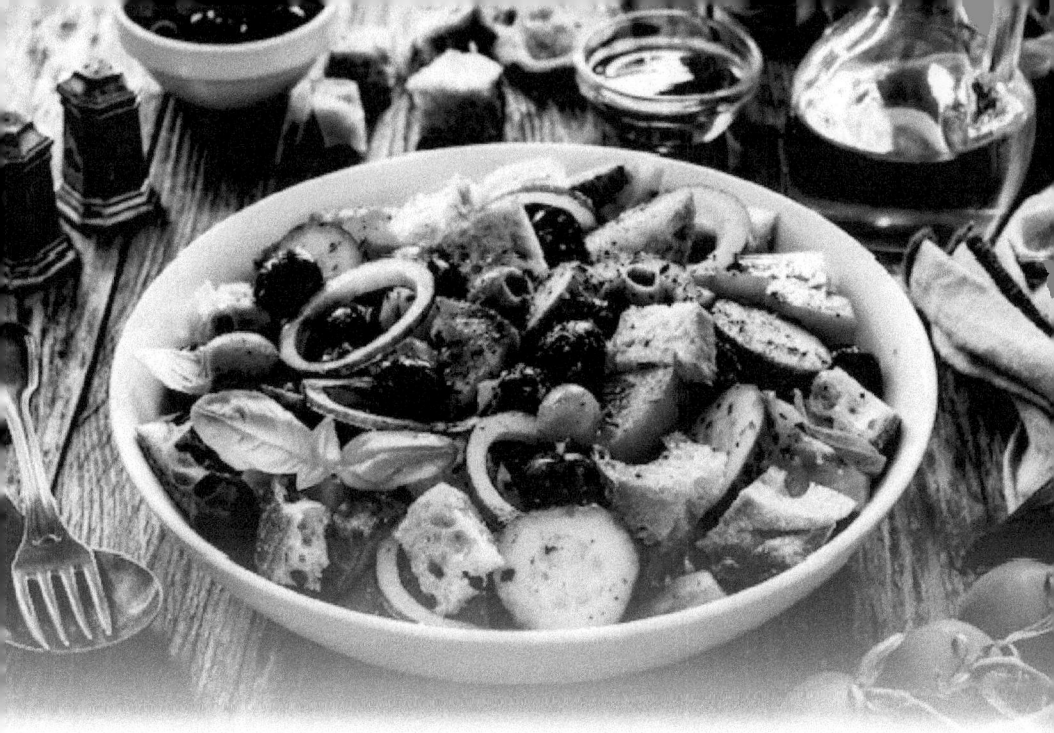

Tuscan Tomato and Bread Salad

6 to 8 servings

INGREDIENTS:

- 1 lb. cherry or grape tomatoes, halved through the stem
- 1lb. fresh mozzarella, 3/4-inch diced
- 2 teaspoons minced garlic
- 1 teaspoon Dijon mustard
- 1/4 cup red wine vinegar
- Salt and freshly ground black pepper
- 1/2 cup plus 1/3 cup olive oil for sautéing bread
- 5 cups sourdough bread, crusts removed and cut into ¾" cubes
- ½ cup fresh basil leaves, julienned

PROCESS:

1. In a large bowl, put in garlic, mustard, vinegar and salt and pepper. Whisk well. Add salt and pepper to taste.

2. Put ½ cup olive oil in a spouted measuring cup. Slowly whisk into vinegar mixture. Set it aside.

3. In a large sauté pan heat 1/3 cup olive oil until hot but not smoking. Add the bread cubes and sprinkle with 1 teaspoon salt and 1/2 teaspoon pepper. Sauté over medium to medium-high heat for 5 to 8 minutes, tossing occasionally, until the bread is evenly browned and crisp.

4. Toss tomatoes and mozzarella with vinaigrette. Add bread cubes and fresh basil. Toss and serve at room temperature.

ACTIVITY – EMBRACE AND LOVE MOVEMENT

Gardening and yard work are fantastic ways to engage in physical activity while nurturing nature and enhancing the beauty of your surroundings. They involve various tasks that work out different muscle groups and boost cardiovascular health. Although my gardening has shifted to container gardening, it still provides a physical workout.

If you don't have a yard, consider volunteering at local gardening projects or community gardens.

Digging and planting:

- Require you to bend, squat, and stretch, which engages your core and leg muscles. The repetitive motions involved in digging can be an effective full-body workout, enhancing flexibility and promoting better posture while also increasing your stamina and strength.

Weeding and Pruning:

- Fantastic for your upper body and requires consistent use of your arms, shoulders, and back, improving muscle strength and endurance. Pruning tall branches may also elevate your heart rate, offering a good cardiovascular workout.

Raking Leaves and Mowing:

- These tasks offer aerobic exercise due to their sustained nature. Raking utilizes large muscle groups, enhancing stamina and coordination. Pushing a lawnmower, whether manual or powered, engages various muscle groups, improving strength and endurance over time.

Watering Plants:

- Especially in a large yard or garden area, this can be physically engaging. Carrying water cans or dragging hose pipes develops arm strength, improves balance, enhances cardiovascular health, and can significantly add to your daily step count.

Gardening and yard work offer the added benefit of fresh air and sunshine, which can help boost your vitamin D levels.

KINDNESS – CULTIVATE IT IN YOUR DAILY LIFE

Volunteering at a senior center is a profoundly rewarding act of kindness. It offers companionship to those who may feel isolated, shares joy through engaging activities, and brings smiles to many faces. Your presence can make a significant impact, reminding seniors that they are valued and loved.

My younger sister has been in assisted living for several years, over 1,000 miles away. I visit as often as I can, as do local family members, and we use Facetime to stay connected. We are very fortunate to have a group of hospice volunteers who regularly stop by to assist with her bathing, sing to her, and even bring her thoughtful gifts like a stuffed kitty that meows.

Make sure to understand these volunteering essentials.

Be patient and compassionate:

- Seniors might move or communicate slower than you're used to. Being patient and kind can make a big difference, creating a supportive and positive environment.

Learn their stories:

- Seniors have a wealth of experiences and stories to share. Take the time to listen, learn from them, and engage in meaningful conversations. Start the conversation by asking straightforward questions such as where they are from.

Offer your skills:

- Whether you have a talent for music, cooking, teaching, or even just good conversation, offer to share your skills and hobbies. Find out what they love to do the most.

Respect their independence:

- While some may need more assistance, others may prefer to do things on their own. Always ask before helping.

Log Today's Activities and Experiences with The SPEAK Method

Use the questions or comments as a guide or write freely expressing your thoughts!

SELF-CARE – How was your nap? How did you feel afterwards? When are you going to take another?

_____
_____
_____
_____
_____
_____
_____
_____

PASSION – List small goals for your passion.

_____
_____
_____
_____
_____
_____
_____
_____

EAT AND ENJOY NOURISHING FOOD – List foods of your season you are going to put on your shopping list.

___

ACTIVITY – If you don't have a garden, do your neighbors need help.

___

KINDNESS – List senior centers in your area and one you will stop by first for volunteering.

_____
_____
_____
_____
_____
_____

ADDITIONAL NOTES

_____
_____
_____
_____
_____
_____

DAILY REPORT CARD OF LIFE – How did you SPEAK today?

Grade Your Day, no D's or F's Allowed!

- **A** – Amazing
- **B** – Better than yesterday
- **C** – Challenging but working on it

DAY 18

> "R-E-S-P-E-C-T Find out what it means to me."
> **Aretha Franklin Iconic Song**

SELF-CARE – PRACTICE IT DAILY

Growing up, "Queen for a Day" was one of my favorite shows. It aired from 1956 to 1964, and I was saddened when it ended. Contestants shared their personal hardships, and the audience would crown a winner, rewarding them with a day of royal treatment. Taking inspiration from this, why not crown yourself "Queen (or King) for a Day" as a unique self-care practice? Imagine a day dedicated entirely to yourself, where you are the sovereign ruler of your own happiness and well-being.

Start Your Royal Day:

- Have a delightful breakfast in bed. Enjoy your favorite morning treats, like freshly squeezed juice, pastries, fruits, and a hot beverage. Take your time savoring each bite while listening to calming music.

Luxurious Spa Experience:

- Transform your bathroom into a personal spa. Draw a warm bubble bath infused with essential oils or bath salts. Light scented candles, play soothing music, and perhaps indulge in a face mask or a body scrub. Let yourself unwind completely.

Personal Shopping Spree:

- Treat yourself to a shopping spree, either online or better yet at your favorite local shops. Buy something special that you've been eyeing, whether it's clothing, accessories, or a unique item that brings you joy.

Private Movie Screening:

- Set up a cozy home theater with your favorite films, snacks, and beverages. Enjoy a marathon of your favorite movies or binge-watch a series you've been wanting to see.

Wear your invisible crown with pride and enjoy a day where you are treated like royalty, because you deserve it.

PASSION – DISCOVER AND IGNITE IT

Finding your passion is a journey that begins with self-reflection and understanding the milestones that have shaped your life. One effective strategy is to conduct a "Passion Audit." This activity involves creating a timeline of your life to highlight significant events, accomplishments, and moments of profound joy. By examining these key points, you'll gain insights into what truly ignites your passion and joy.

Where Were You?

- Identify the locations where these significant moments occurred. Whether it was your childhood home, a particular city, or a memorable travel destination, understanding the environment can provide context to your experience.

Who were you with?

- Consider the people who shared these moments with you. Friends, family members, mentors, or even strangers may have played a role in your happiest and most formative experiences. Their influence can highlight the types of relationships that support your passion.

How old were you?

- Pinpointing your age during these events can help you see patterns over different life stages. It might reveal how your interests have evolved or remained consistent, helping you understand the core elements of your passion.

What was significant?

- Reflect on why these moments were meaningful to you. Was it an achievement, a personal breakthrough, or a simple yet impactful experience? Identifying the essence of what made these times joyful will bring clarity to your true passions.

This self-discovery process will guide you towards a life filled with purpose and enthusiasm, aligned with what you are truly passionate about.

EAT AND ENJOY – NOURISHING FOOD

Creating your own salad dressings is a delightful way to enhance your meals with fresh, flavorful ingredients. They are quick and easy to make, save money, and avoid the preservatives and additives found in store-bought versions. Start with the basics: choose a healthy oil and combine it with an acid, such as any type of vinegar or lemon juice.

Salad Dressing in a Jar:

- Vinaigrettes are perfect for this method. Simply add all ingredients to a jar, seal it tightly, and shake well. This effortless technique ensures a well-mixed, delicious dressing every time. I recycle all my glass jars to use for making and storing dressings.

Make Healthy Versions:

- Salad dressings can seem healthy but often contain hidden sugars and unhealthy oils. When making your own, choose olive or avocado oil and sweeten with natural options like honey, maple syrup, or monk fruit. Enjoy my famous **Ranch Dressing and Dip**.

Explore Global Flavors:

- Try an Asian Vinaigrette with rice vinegar, soy sauce, ginger and olive oil. Use salsa to make a quick Mexican dressing with avocado oil and lemon juice. Create an Italian dressing with red wine vinegar, olive oil and Italian Seasoning.

Experiment with Infused Oils and Vinegars:

- Explore specialty shops for vinegars infused with garlic, fig, orange, or other unique flavors. Additionally, try flavored olive oils such as rosemary, basil, or truffle. You can also experiment with infusing your own oils.

Homemade dressings are quick and easy to make. Enjoy experimenting with different combinations to create unique flavors.

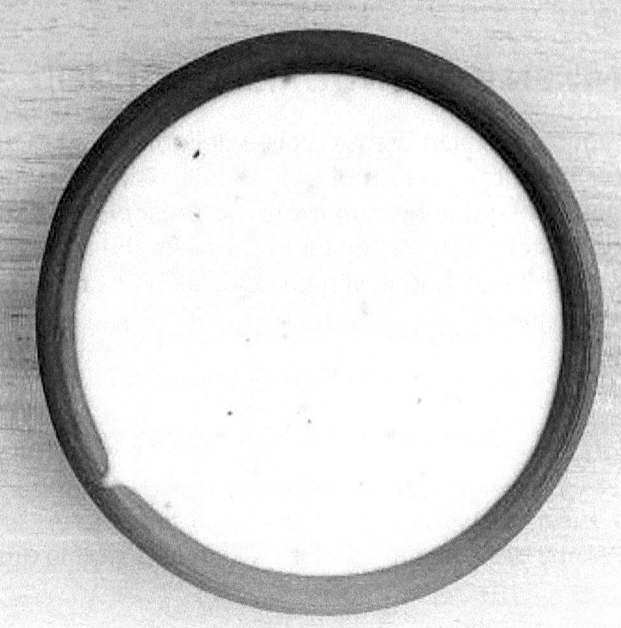

Ranch Dressing and Dip

Ranch Dressing Powder Mixture:

INGREDIENTS:

- 1/2 cup dry buttermilk powder
- 2 Tablespoons dried parsley flakes
- 1 teaspoon dried dill weed
- 1 teaspoon dried onion flakes
- 1 teaspoon onion powder
- 2 teaspoon garlic powder
- 1 teaspoon sea salt
- 1/4 teaspoon ground pepper
- 1/2 teaspoon powdered monk fruit or stevia

PROCESS:

1. Put everything in a bowl and mix.
2. RECOMMENDED: To have a finer powder and consistent mixture, put all ingredients in a food processor or blender and pulse once or twice just to incorporate.

3. Store in a jar with a tight-fitting lid. Use it in any recipe that requires a packet of ranch dressing.
4. One packet is 2 1/2 Tablespoons of the above mixture.

Ranch Dressing INGREDIENTS:

- 1 cup mayonnaise, sugar free
- 1/2 cup Greek yogurt
- 1/4 cup milk mixed with 1 teaspoon cider vinegar and allowed to sit for 10 minutes (this makes a buttermilk)
- 2 1/2 Tablespoons Ranch Dressing Powder Mix

PROCESS:

1. Combine dressing ingredients in a bowl and whisk until smooth.
2. Store in jar in the refrigerator for 2 weeks.

ACTIVITY – EMBRACE AND LOVE MOVEMENT

Parking farther away from your destination can be an easy and effective way to integrate more physical activity into your daily routine. This small change can lead to significant health benefits and improve your overall well-being. By making this conscious choice, you also foster a more active lifestyle and set a positive example for others. Remember safety first when on your own or parking after dark.

Increased Daily Steps:

- By parking further from your destination, you naturally add more steps to your day. This can help you reach and surpass your daily step goals, contributing to improved cardiovascular health and stamina.

Enhanced Calorie Burn:

- Walking those extra few minutes each day can contribute to a higher calorie burn, aiding in weight management. Even short bursts of extra activity can add up over time to help maintain a healthy weight and improve metabolism.

Mental Health Boost:

- By parking farther away, you give yourself the opportunity for a short walk that can help reduce stress, improve mood, provide a mental break from your busy schedule, and promote mindfulness by allowing you to enjoy your surroundings.

Environmental Impact:

- Parking farther away can also have a positive environmental impact. By reducing the time you spend circling for a close parking spot, you cut down on fuel consumption and minimize vehicle emissions, contributing to a greener environment.

Incorporating this simple habit into your daily routine can enhance both your physical health and your overall quality of life.

KINDNESS – CULTIVATE IT IN YOUR DAILY LIFE

Respecting others is one of the simplest yet most profound acts of kindness we can offer. It fosters an environment where everyone feels valued and heard, encouraging openness and trust.

Being Punctual:

- Valuing other people's time by being punctual is a clear sign of respect. It shows that you are considerate of their schedule and commitments, and it helps to build trust and reliability in any relationship. I have a habit of telling friends or family who are always late that we're starting half an hour earlier than we are. Oops, I gave my trick away!

Cultural Sensitivity:

- Respecting Individuals from different cultural backgrounds means being open and considerate of their customs, traditions, and beliefs. Take the time to learn and understand these differences and embrace the diversity they bring to our lives.

Using Polite and Respectful Language:

- The words we choose matter. Using polite and respectful language, avoiding derogatory terms, and speaking kindly can help maintain a respectful atmosphere. Even when differences arise, constructive and respectful dialogue is key.

Being Supportive and Encouraging:

- Offer support and encouragement to others, especially during challenging times. By being a positive presence and offering words of encouragement, you show that you respect their journey and believe in their abilities.

By incorporating these respectful behaviors into our daily lives, we contribute positively to the wellbeing of those around us, promoting a kind and empathetic community.

Log Today's Activities and Experiences with The SPEAK Method

Use the questions or comments as a guide or write freely expressing your thoughts!

SELF-CARE – When is your next "Queen or King for a Day"? What are your plans?

_____
_____
_____
_____
_____
_____

PASSION – Write down your Passion Audit. What are the particulars?

_____
_____
_____
_____
_____
_____
_____

EAT AND ENJOY NOURISHING FOOD – List your favorite salad dressings. How are you going to make them healthy and what new ones are you excited to try?

ACTIVITY – What stores are you going to park farther away from?

KINDNESS – What steps do you take to respect others?

_____
_____
_____
_____
_____
_____

ADDITIONAL NOTES

_____
_____
_____
_____
_____
_____

DAILY REPORT CARD OF LIFE – How did you SPEAK today?

Grade Your Day, no D's or F's Allowed!

- **A** – Amazing
- **B** – Better than yesterday
- **C** – Challenging but working on it

Interview
Sheng Belmonte

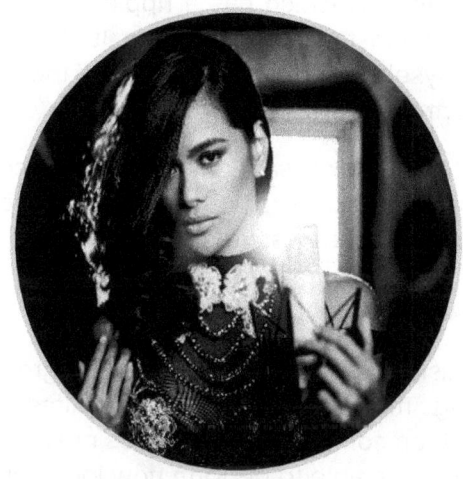

- Miss Fitspiration Philippines 2018,
- Recording Artist with Sony Music Philippines 2010 – 2011. Debut album (EP) "Sheng Belmonte" - Nominated for Best New Female Artist of the Year and Best Music Video.
- Recording Artist and Actress with Viva Records and Viva Artist Agency 2012-2017. Song, "Single"- Nominated as Best Dance Song of the Year. Performed in TV, movie and acting projects.
- During the pandemic in 2022 released my first self-produced song and Music Video called "Let Me Know" and was nominated for Hollywood Independent Music Awards under Dance Music category.

SELF-CARE – PRACTICE IT DAILY

Self-care has always been important to me, and I've found that my approach to it has evolved, especially during this challenging period in my life. Some of my favorite self-care activities include meditation, fitness or any form of movement, listening to or watching self-development podcasts, and creating healthier versions of my favorite foods.

Finding time for self-care in my current situation requires creativity and flexibility. For example, I often listen to podcasts or interviews that help me improve my mindset while getting ready for work or during my commute. This practice rewires my brain to think more positively about myself, which has a ripple effect on how I view others and the circumstances I encounter. It also encourages me to be kinder to myself, which I believe is one of the most consistent and effective forms of self-care.

By letting go of the unnecessary guilt that often accompanies prioritizing self-care—especially for women—I'm able to build my self-worth and show up as the best version of myself.

PASSION – DISCOVER AND IGNITE IT

Singing and music will always be one of my greatest passions. Performing brings me a sense of joy and fulfillment that's hard to replicate. It's a deep connection that makes me feel alive and I am grateful that I've been able to perform now locally in Minnesota.

Since moving to the U.S., my interests have expanded and evolved in meaningful ways.

I have always been driven to inspire others through my personal health and fitness journey, as well as my mindset transformations. This has evolved into a strong interest in understanding the science of how our bodies work and change as we age and how our thoughts shape our reality. Additionally, I've found a growing interest in entrepreneurship, which I believe has been influenced by my husband. While I was an artist in the entertainment industry, I had management and labels take care of the business side. Then, during the peak of my career, things moved so fast that I didn't have the chance to fully grasp the business aspects. I am now passionate about developing my business and leadership skills to support future artists and brands.

EAT AND ENJOY - NOURISHING FOOD

Coming from a big family with six children, we had very humble beginnings. Instant noodles and canned foods were staples, often divided into small portions to feed everyone. When I started living on my own and traveling around Asia to perform with my band at the age of 18, my diet didn't improve much—I mostly relied on fried foods or ready-to-eat microwavable meals.

At 26, I became a reality show TV personality and, at 29, a signed artist, embarking on my journey toward a healthy lifestyle. Maintaining a fit and conditioned body became essential, not just for the strength and endurance to sing and dance on stage, but also to manage the demands of a busy schedule.

I discovered that proper nutrition, not just "dieting", and consistent body training were key to achieving my healthiest self, which naturally translated into looking my best for my age. Over time, especially in my mid-30s, I also realized the crucial role that mindset plays in eating and overall wellness.

ACTIVITY – EMBRACE AND LOVE MOVEMENT

In today's fast paced social media era, it's easy to see young people who seem to have endless time and energy to spend at the gym. While this might initially "inspire" others to get into fitness, it can also leave many feeling stuck in the "only ifs..."—only if I had the time, the energy, or the youth.

I believe the best way to inspire people today is by being relatable. I want them to know that I'm just like them—I face struggles too, from the responsibilities that come with midlife to the natural changes in my body. By sharing the simple adjustments that I make in my own life to overcome these challenges, I hope to show that fitness is achievable for everyone, no matter their age or circumstances. It's about finding activities that bring joy and fit into your current lifestyle. For example, I count wrestling with my stepson as a workout because there are days when I wake up sore from it; I get in some movement while also bonding with him.

I also consistently encourage women to lift weights. Building muscle not only enhances our appearance by creating a toned look but also plays a crucial role in fat-burning and longevity.

KINDNESS – CULTIVATE IT IN YOUR DAILY LIFE

I'm grateful to have parents who always emphasized doing the right thing. They instilled in me the belief that kindness is not just a virtue but a way of life. My mom often spoke about karma.

Whenever someone treated her unkindly, she would simply say, "Let karma be the judge," trusting that good and bad deeds eventually come full circle. She believed that when you do good, good things will come back to you.

As I've grown older, I've come to understand that beyond karma, there's a deeper reward in being kind. It feels inherently good to do the right thing and to treat others with kindness. My parents' teachings have shaped my belief that kindness isn't just about what you get in return—it's about the positive impact it has on your own heart and on the world around you.

Website: https://www.shengbelmonte.com

Youtube: https://www.youtube.com/@ShengBelmonteOfficial

Facebook: https://www.facebook.com/thefitsingershengb/

Spotify: https://open.spotify.com/playlist/09xiJe2dQrn5m5gScBQX2O?si=b1c32f9af65e4a3a

Contact : sheng@shengbelmonte.com

DAY 19

> "I play my best when I'm having fun. When you love what you do, and you're out there enjoying it, that's when you're at your best."
> **Caitlin Clark, Iowa Hawkeye and WNBA Basketball Star**

SELF-CARE – PRACTICE IT DAILY

Staying connected with family and friends is crucial for self-care. During the pandemic, physical isolation forced us to rely on technology to maintain our connections. This shift often led to feelings of depression and anxiety. Prioritizing meaningful interactions helps maintain strong relationships.

Schedule Regular Catch Ups:

- Set aside specific times each week or month to catch up with loved ones. Whether through phone calls, video chats, or better yet, in-person visits, consistent communication helps maintain and strengthen your relationships. Don't assume the person is too busy to connect.

Engage in Shared Activities:

- Find hobbies or activities you both enjoy and engage in them together. My favorites include enjoying live music and cooking together with friends. Yours could be book clubs or game nights. Shared experiences create lasting bonds.

Express Appreciation:

- Regularly tell your friends and family how much they mean to you. Send handwritten notes, thoughtful texts, or small gifts to show your gratitude. End a phone call or a text with "I appreciate you."

Personal Updates:

- Frequently check in with your friends and family to see what they've been up to. Refer to topics from previous conversations and share your own life updates or projects. Even simple topics, like how your garden is doing, can foster connection. My brother and I often discuss our tomato plants; he was even featured on a gardening magazine cover for his tomatoes.

Incorporating time with loved ones into your self-care routine is a valuable reminder that support, and joy are always within reach.

PASSION – DISCOVER AND IGNITE IT

The importance of having fun in activities you're passionate about often gets overlooked. While every passionate pursuit will have its challenging days, the fun should outweigh them. My favorite sports star, Caitlin Clark, exemplifies this balance. Even during tough games, she ends with a smile and has fun signing autographs for kids. Passion and fun should always go hand in hand.

Set Small, Attainable Goals:

- This is a powerful way to keep the journey enjoyable and prevent it from becoming overwhelming. When you set smaller goals, you give yourself more opportunities to celebrate achievements.

Incorporate Playfulness:

- Bringing a sense of playfulness into your passion can transform your experience and keep your enthusiasm alive. When you approach your pursuits with a lighthearted and playful attitude, you open the door to creativity, innovation, and enjoy the process rather than being solely focused on the outcome.

Stay Connected with Fun People:

- Surrounding yourself with people who bring joy, laughter, and positivity into your life can elevate your passion to new heights. When you're around individuals who not only share your interests but also know how to have a good time, it creates an environment where creativity thrives.

Mix Things Up:

- Keeping your passion fresh and exciting is key to maintaining long-term enjoyment. One of the best ways to achieve this is by mixing things up. By introducing variety and trying new approaches, you prevent boredom and make the journey more fun and invigorating.

Go ahead and have fun doing what you love.

EAT AND ENJOY – NOURISHING FOOD

Nature often provides clues about the health benefits of food. As a child, I wasn't fond of carrots, but my mom always said, "Eat your carrots; they're good for your eyes." Later, I realized that my mom was smart; sliced carrots resemble the iris of the eye.

Tomatoes:

- With their heart-like appearance, tomatoes are a perfect example of nature's signatures. When you cut open a tomato, you'll notice it resembles the chambers of the heart. They are rich in lycopene, an antioxidant that supports heart health.

Walnuts:

- Encased in a shell resembling a skull, cracked open walnuts reveal two "hemispheres" inside akin to your brain structure. These "brain-like" nuts are rich in omega-3 fatty acids, supporting cognitive function and brain health.

Bananas:

- With their curved shape, bananas resemble the muscles in our arms, High in potassium, they aid in muscle function and help maintain proper electrolyte balance, making them a perfect natural energy booster. Try my delicious **Banana Walnut Bread**.

Avocados:

- Avocados are my favorite signature of nature. During my time in Panama, I had an avocado tree and discovered that it takes nine months for the fruit to mature from flower to ripe avocado. Cut open an avocado, observe its resemblance to the womb of a pregnant woman, with the seed as the developing baby. Avocados are packed with healthy fatty acids that support hormonal and cardiovascular health.

Like my mom, nature is also smart, start your 'signatures of nature search' and you will be amazed.

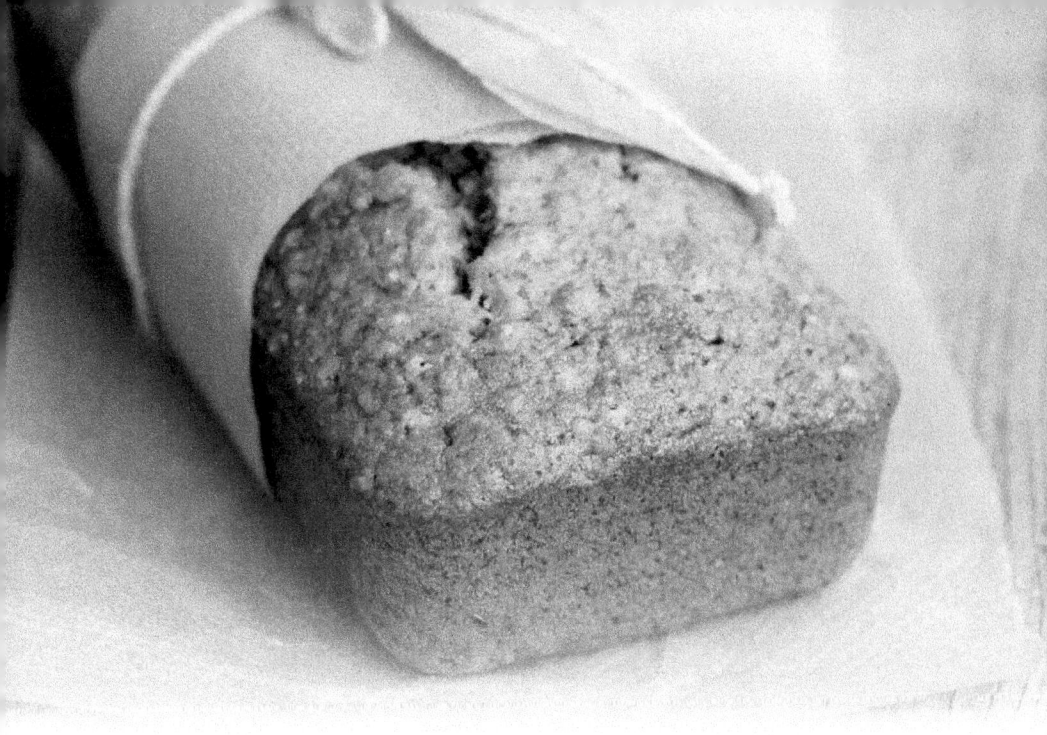

Banana Walnut Bread

6-8 Servings

INGREDIENTS:

- 3 ripe bananas, mashed
- 1/3 cup honey
- 1/4 cup melted coconut oil or butter
- 1 large egg, beaten
- 1 teaspoon vanilla extract
- 1 teaspoon baking soda
- A pinch of salt
- 1 1/2 cups white whole wheat flour or gluten free blend
- 1/2 cup chopped walnuts

PROCESS:

1. Preheat oven to 350°F
2. Grease a 9x5-inch loaf pan.
3. In a large mixing bowl, combine the mashed bananas, honey, melted coconut oil (or butter), beaten egg, and vanilla extract. Stir until smooth.

4. In a separate bowl, mix the baking soda, salt, and flour together.
5. Gradually add the dry ingredients to the wet mixture, stirring just until combined. Be careful not to overmix.
6. Gently fold in the chopped walnuts until evenly distributed.
7. Pour the batter into the prepared loaf pan. Bake for 50-60 minutes, or until a toothpick inserted into the center comes out clean.
8. Let bread cool in the pan for 10 minutes before transferring it to a wire rack to cool completely.

ACTIVITY – EMBRACE AND LOVE MOVEMENT

Jumping rope is an activity from childhood that we rarely continue as adults. In Panama, we lived next door to a family with a young girl who loved to jump rope. She enticed me to join her. Although I wasn't as fast as I used to be, I was able to show her some old tricks. Get a jump rope and try some simple movements.

Selecting a Jump Rope:

- Choose a rope that is appropriate for your height. When you stand on the middle of the rope, the handles should reach your armpits. Opt for a lightweight and durable rope for easier handling and consider a beaded or segmented rope if you are a beginner.

Start Small:

- Begin with short sessions of just a few minutes each day, gradually increasing the time and intensity as you become more comfortable. This helps build stamina and reduces the risk of injury. You can even start by twirling the rope overhead and walking over it rather than jumping. Every little bit of movement helps.

Protect Your Joints:

- To minimize joint stress, always jump on a soft surface like a gym mat or grassy area. Wear supportive athletic shoes with good cushioning, and focus on low-impact jumps, keeping them small and controlled.

Warm-Up and Cool Down:

- Incorporate a proper warm-up before you start jumping rope, including stretches and light cardio. After your session, perform static stretches to cool down and aid in muscle recovery.

The key is to have fun and rekindle fond memories of your youth.

KINDNESS – CULTIVATE IT IN YOUR DAILY LIFE

Start a Positivity Chain by creating a group text or social media thread where everyone shares recent positive experiences or fun activities. This simple initiative can uplift spirits, foster connections, and encourage a ripple effect of goodness in your community. By sharing fun moments of joy, gratitude, and kindness, we can create a supportive environment where everyone feels valued and inspired. Let's come together to make our community a beacon of hope and happiness.

Share a Positive Pet Experience and Picture:

- Post a heartwarming pic of your furry friend, sharing a moment that brought you joy. Pets have a magical way of lifting our spirits with their unconditional love

Share great meal:

- Showcase a delicious meal you cooked or savored at a restaurant. Describe the flavors and experience, inspiring others with culinary delight and the joy of good food. Be sure to add a picture.

Share an Enjoyable Event:

- Highlight a special event, concert, or a serene day at the beach. Capture the essence of the moment to spread happiness and remind others of life's simple pleasures.

Share an Old Picture:

- Post a nostalgic photo that brings back fond memories. Denote when and where it was taken and why it makes you smile. Whether it's a childhood moment or a fun past adventure, sharing this can brighten someone's day.

Join in the positivity chain and watch as our collective efforts create a wave of positive change!

Log Today's Activities and Experiences with The SPEAK Method

Use the questions or comments as a guide or write freely expressing your thoughts!

SELF-CARE – Who have you re-connected with today and who is on your connection list?

_____
_____
_____
_____
_____
_____
_____
_____

PASSION – How do you plan to incorporate fun with your passion?

_____
_____
_____
_____
_____
_____
_____
_____

EAT AND ENJOY NOURISHING FOOD – What 'signatures of nature' did you identify?

_____
_____
_____
_____
_____
_____
_____
_____

ACTIVITY – Did you order a jumping rope, or do you already have one?

_____
_____
_____
_____
_____
_____
_____
_____

KINDNESS – Where did you start the positivity chain?

_____
_____
_____
_____
_____

ADDITIONAL NOTES

_____
_____
_____
_____
_____

DAILY REPORT CARD OF LIFE – How did you SPEAK today?

Grade Your Day, no D's or F's Allowed!

- **A** – Amazing
- **B** – Better than yesterday
- **C** – Challenging but working on it

DAY 20

> "We need four hugs a day for survival. We need eight hugs a day for maintenance. We need twelve hugs a day for growth."
> **Virginia Satir**

SELF-CARE – PRACTICE IT DAILY

Hugs are one of the most important self-care actions. Many years ago, I had the pleasure of attending a conference in Maui. Although it was a business conference, one of the speakers emphasized the significance of hugs for both mental and physical health. This was probably the best part of the conference as everybody was hugging!

Why Hug:

- Hugs reduce stress, foster deeper connections, and boost mood through the release of oxytocin, the love hormone. Hugs also lower blood pressure, promote heart health, and provide a sense of security and comfort.

How to Hug:

- A heart-to-heart hug aligns the left sides of two people, connecting their hearts. This nurturing embrace fosters deeper emotional bonds, synchronizes heartbeats, and creates a profound sense of unity and comfort. Youngsters naturally love to hug, so teach them the heart-to-heart method early on.

When to Hug:

- Anytime! Not really but be sure to hug when greeting friends and family. Hug during moments of joy like birthdays, anniversaries, or achievements. Hug when someone is feeling sad or going through a tough time. Hug after an argument or disagreement to show forgiveness.

Who to Hug:

- Almost everyone! Always be mindful of personal space. While some people, like my husband, are natural huggers, others might prefer more distance, and that's perfectly okay. In that case, make it a gentle embrace.

Embrace the power of hugs in your daily routine to nurture yourself and cultivate a deeper bond with those around you.

PASSION – DISCOVER AND IGNITE IT

At my favorite brother-in-law's funeral, his youngest daughter delivered the eulogy. Reflecting on her words, she recounted his passions, from his devotion to the Minnesota Vikings to his joy in teasing kids with his Donald Duck voice. Take some time to write your own eulogy; it will help you uncover and ignite your passions before it's too late.

Personal Qualities and Character:

- List your unique traits and characteristics that made you special. What are your values and how have you impacted others positively? Consider instances where your kindness or leadership made a difference.

Memorable Stories and Anecdotes:

- Share specific stories or moments that exemplify your character and the way you have lived. What are some funny things people remember about you? Highlight the times when your humor brought joy to others.

Achievements and Passions:

- List your significant accomplishments, hobbies, or passions and why they are important to you. This can include career achievements, community involvement, personal interests, and the impact these pursuits have had on your life and others.

Impact on Others:

- Reflect on the ways you have touched the lives of family, friends, and the community. Talk about your relationships, acts of kindness, and the legacy you want to leave behind. Share memories of meaningful connections, selfless deeds, and the positive impact you have made on others.

Writing your own eulogy not only allows you to reflect on your life's journey but also helps ignite your passion by reaffirming the values and goals that matter most to you.

EAT AND ENJOY – NOURISHING FOOD

Food plays a critical role not only in fueling our bodies but also in significantly influencing our mood and emotional well-being. By making mindful dietary choices, we can harness the power of food to improve our mental health and cultivate a more positive state of mind.

Salmon and Other Oily Fish:

- Rich in omega-3 fatty acids, salmon, mackerel, and sardines support brain health and function. They have also been linked to reduced symptoms of depression and anxiety. Try grilled, baked, sautéed or salmon cakes.

Sweet Potatoes:

- Nothing says comfort food like sweet potatoes. Packed with complex carbohydrates, they provide a steady release of glucose into the bloodstream, preventing energy crashes and mood swings. Growing up, we always enjoyed sweet potato casserole topped with mini marshmallows for Thanksgiving. Now, my new family favorite **is Pecan Sweet Potato Casserole.**

Nuts:

- Incorporating nuts like almonds, pecans and walnuts that are rich in magnesium can reduce symptoms of depression and anxiety. Add nuts to yogurt, oatmeal, and a salad or have as a snack. Remember to watch portion size, it is easy to lose track while eating that can of nuts.

Beans:

- Kidney beans, black beans, chickpeas, lentils and other beans are excellent sources of protein and fiber. They help stabilize blood sugar levels, reducing mood swings. They also contain B vitamins, which are essential for mood regulation. For a salty snack, try roasted chickpea crisps.

Incorporating these mood-boosting foods into your diet can help you feel more balanced, energized, and happy.

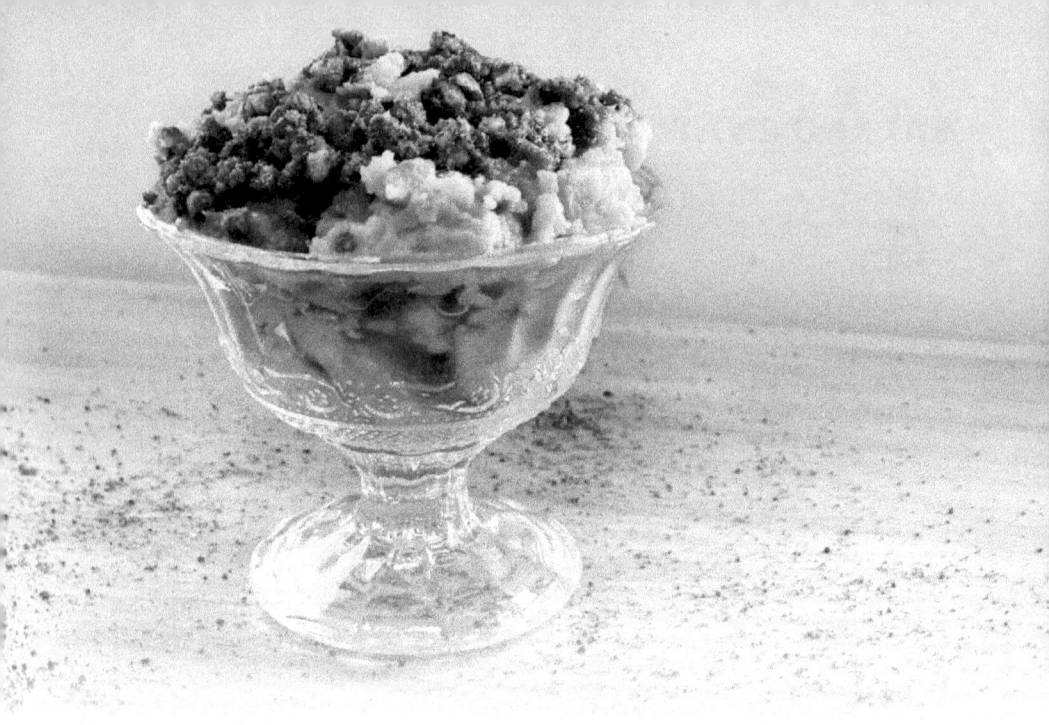

Pecan Sweet Potato Casserole

8-10 Servings

INGREDIENTS:

- 6 cups sweet potatoes, peeled and cubed
- 1/2 cup honey
- 3 eggs, beaten
- 3 Tablespoons butter
- 3/4 cup unsweetened almond milk
- 1 teaspoon vanilla
- 1 teaspoon sea salt

TOPPING:

- 1/3 cup coconut sugar
- 1/3 cup whole wheat or gluten free flour
- 3 Tablespoons butter, softened
- 1/2 cup pecan pieces
- 1 teaspoon cinnamon

Combine the above topping ingredients in a small bowl and mix with a fork to crumble.

PROCESS:

1. Preheat oven to 325°F.
2. Put sweet potatoes in a medium saucepan with water to cover.
3. Cook over medium high heat until tender; drain and mash.
4. In a large bowl, beat eggs and add cooked potatoes, honey, salt, butter, milk and vanilla.
5. Using a hand mixer, beat until smooth.
6. Transfer to an oiled 9x13 inch baking dish.
7. Top with topping.
8. Bake in preheated oven for 30 minutes or until topping is browned.

ACTIVITY – EMBRACE AND LOVE MOVEMENT

As I mentioned earlier, water is my element when it comes to embracing movement. The buoyancy provided by water reduces the impact on joints, making it an ideal option for people of all ages and fitness levels. Whether you prefer the pool, the ocean, or a lake, there are various water-based movements to try.

Water Aerobics:

- Involves performing aerobic routines in shallow or deep water. Water aerobics classes often include a mix of cardio, strength training, and flexibility exercises. The resistance provided by water helps tone muscles while being gentle on the joints.

Jogging in Water:

- Also known as aqua jogging, this exercise can be performed in both shallow and deep water. Jogging in water increases cardiovascular endurance and muscle strength while minimizing joint strain.

Kick Board or Boogie Boarding:

- Using a kickboard or boogie board can turn a day at the beach or pool into a fun core and leg workout.

    My husband and I have been fortunate to go boogie boarding in Panama, Costa Rica, Hawaii, and off the beaches near our home in North Carolina, South Carolina, Georgia and Florida. I vote Panama as the best!

Water Bicycling:

- While floating on your back, use a pool noodle for support and mimic cycling motions with your legs. This low-resistance exercise targets your lower body and core, enhancing flexibility.

Integrating water exercises into your fitness routine can help you stay active and healthy while adding a fun twist to your regular workouts.

KINDNESS – CULTIVATE IT IN YOUR DAILY LIFE

Sharing is a selfless act of kindness that fosters strong connections, spreads joy, and enhances the sense of community among individuals. By sharing knowledge, resources, and experiences, we create a supportive environment that uplifts and strengthens the bonds between people.

Recipes:

- As a chef, I love to share recipes. Also, asking someone for a recipe makes them feel valued. BONUS: This month, enjoy an extra recipe— **Ultimate Pasta Salad** shared by my dear friend and fantastic cook, Ann.

Local Events:

- Sharing information about local events is a simple yet impactful act of kindness. Share festivals, local markets, favorite shops, fairs, or music events. Many of my friends are big fans of live music, and our area offers plenty of free concerts. I make sure to let them know when our favorite bands are playing, plus we get the bonus of exercise while dancing!

Shops and Restaurants:

- As a "foodie," I love sharing new restaurants or places where I've had great food. Also, suggest your favorite local shops. I once shared my favorite boutique with a friend, and she became a loyal customer. This act of kindness also supports local businesses.

Book Recommendations:

- Recommend your latest reads or must-read classics. If a friend travels frequently, share an audiobook to help them pass the time. When sharing a book, consider their interests to make it more meaningful. Sharing a favorite read on social media creates an uplifting post.

Spread joy sharing a few of your favorite things.

Ultimate Pasta Salad

8-10 Servings

SALAD INGREDIENTS:

- 1 lb. penne or fusilli pasta, cooked al dente. HINT: Drain and rinse with cold water until cool. Shake off excess water, then toss with 1Tablespoon olive oil
- 1 cup fire-roasted red peppers, rinsed and rough chopped
- ½ cup artichoke hearts, rinsed and chopped
- 12 oz. smoked gouda, cubed
- 3 Tablespoons fresh parsley, rough chopped
- 3 Tablespoons fresh basil, rough chopped

DRESSING INGREDIENTS:

- ½ cup mayonnaise or plain Greek yogurt (try ¼ cup of each)
- ¼ cup olive oil
- 2 Tablespoons white wine vinegar
- 2 cloves garlic, finely minced
- 2 teaspoons honey
- 1 teaspoon adobe sauce from canned chipotle peppers
- 1 teaspoon salt
- Fresh ground pepper to taste

PROCESS:

1. In a large bowl, combine mayonnaise and/or yogurt, olive oil, garlic, honey, adobe sauce, salt and pepper.
2. Whisk until smooth.
3. Add cooked pasta, peppers, artichoke hearts, gouda, parsley and basil.
4. Gently toss to combine.
5. Cover and store in refrigerator for 4-6 hours or overnight.
6. Let rest at room temperature 15-20 minutes before serving. This thickens the dressing. Stir before serving.

Log Today's Activities and Experiences with The SPEAK Method

Use the questions or comments as a guide or write freely expressing your thoughts!

SELF-CARE – List the people you have hugged today.

PASSION – List the things you would talk about in your eulogy.

EAT AND ENJOY NOURISHING FOOD – How does food influence your food? List some mood improving foods to try.

_____
_____
_____
_____
_____
_____
_____
_____

ACTIVITY – What water activities do you enjoy and what ones do you have planned?

_____
_____
_____
_____
_____
_____
_____
_____

KINDNESS – List things you are going to share.

_____
_____
_____
_____
_____
_____

ADDITIONAL NOTES

_____
_____
_____
_____
_____
_____

DAILY REPORT CARD OF LIFE – How did you SPEAK today?

Grade Your Day, no D's or F's Allowed!

- **A** – Amazing
- **B** – Better than yesterday
- **C** – Challenging but working on it

DAY 21

"Solitude is where I place my chaos to rest and awaken my inner peace."
Nikki Rowe

SELF-CARE – PRACTICE IT DAILY

Enjoy your own company and do something you truly love without needing anyone else to join. Be sure to stay off social media to fully immerse yourself in the experience.

Solo Dining Date:

- Start your day with coffee and breakfast at a cozy café, savoring your favorite beverage and a good book. Or have dinner at your favorite restaurant's bar area to easily engage with fellow customers or the bartender, making new friends along the way.

Stroll a Local Museum or Art Gallery:

- Immerse yourself in the creativity and history of the exhibits. Explore at your own pace and take the time to appreciate the details that captivate you most. Allow yourself to truly connect with the art and history around you.

Treat Yourself to a Picnic:

- Find a safe area in a nearby park. Pack a healthy and delicious lunch, a soft blanket, and perhaps a favorite magazine. After your meal, allow yourself to unwind with a relaxing nap under the open sky.

Attend Events:

- Enjoy watching a movie at the theater, attending a play, or experiencing a local live music performance. Laugh at the funny movies, cry at the sad ones, and dance like nobody's watching at the live music events.

Spending time alone and engaging in activities you love will rejuvenate your spirit and foster a deeper connection with yourself.

PASSION – DISCOVER AND IGNITE IT

Ask Yourself 5 'Why' Questions: Start with a broad question about something that interests you and keep asking "why" until you reach a deeper understanding of what drives you. This technique will help surface underlying motivations and values that define your passion.

Why does it fascinate me?

- Does it inspire creative ideas and innovative thinking? Does it present challenges that encourage growth, skill development, and endless learning opportunities, offering a sense of accomplishment? Does it resonate deeply with past experiences or memories, creating a strong emotional connection?

Why do I feel happy or fulfilled?

- Do I feel a shift in my mood or energy when I discuss or engage in this interest? Have friends or family mentioned observing a change in my mood when it comes up? What emotions do I experience before, during, and after engaging in this interest?

Why is it important for me to invest time and energy?

- How does it align with my values? How does this interest enhance my day-to-day life? What benefits do I gain from it? Does it challenge me to learn and grow? Does it help me connect with others?

Why do I prefer it over other activities?

- What unique satisfaction does it provide? How does it align with my personal strengths? In what ways does it fulfill my emotional and creative needs? Does it offer unparalleled joy and excitement?

Understanding your deepest motivations and values through this simple yet profound exercise can illuminate the core of what truly drives you.

EAT AND ENJOY – NOURISHING FOOD

We all have our international food favorites. Mine is a toss-up between Thai and Italian. By using wholesome ingredients and mindful cooking techniques, you can enjoy the rich flavors of global cuisines while maintaining a balanced diet.

Italian:

- Transform classic dishes like chicken parmesan by using gluten free breadcrumbs and whole grain pasta. Substitute heavy cream with a lighter alternative like cream cheese and chicken broth. Enjoy Bolognese made with lean proteins such as ground chicken or turkey. Even kids love the crispy chicken used to make **Chicken Parmesan.**

Thai:

- Enjoy the vibrant flavors of Thai cuisine by making fresh spring rolls rather than fried ones. Create your own Pad Thai sauce with reduced sugar content and sweeten traditional peanut sauce with monk fruit. Pack your dishes with colorful veggies and your choice of tofu, chicken, or shrimp.

Mexican:

- Make your favorite Mexican fare more nourishing by preparing tacos with corn or whole grain tortillas and filling them with grilled fish, chicken, black beans, and plenty of fresh salsa and avocado. Swap sour cream for a dollop of plain Greek yogurt to add creaminess without the extra calories.

Mediterranean:

- Craft a hearty Mediterranean meal by building a balanced plate with cauliflower rice, roasted vegetables, and a generous serving of tzatziki and hummus. Add in some grilled chicken kebobs or falafel for protein, and drizzle with olive oil and lemon juice.

These nourishing takes on international favorites prove that you don't have to sacrifice flavor to eat healthily.

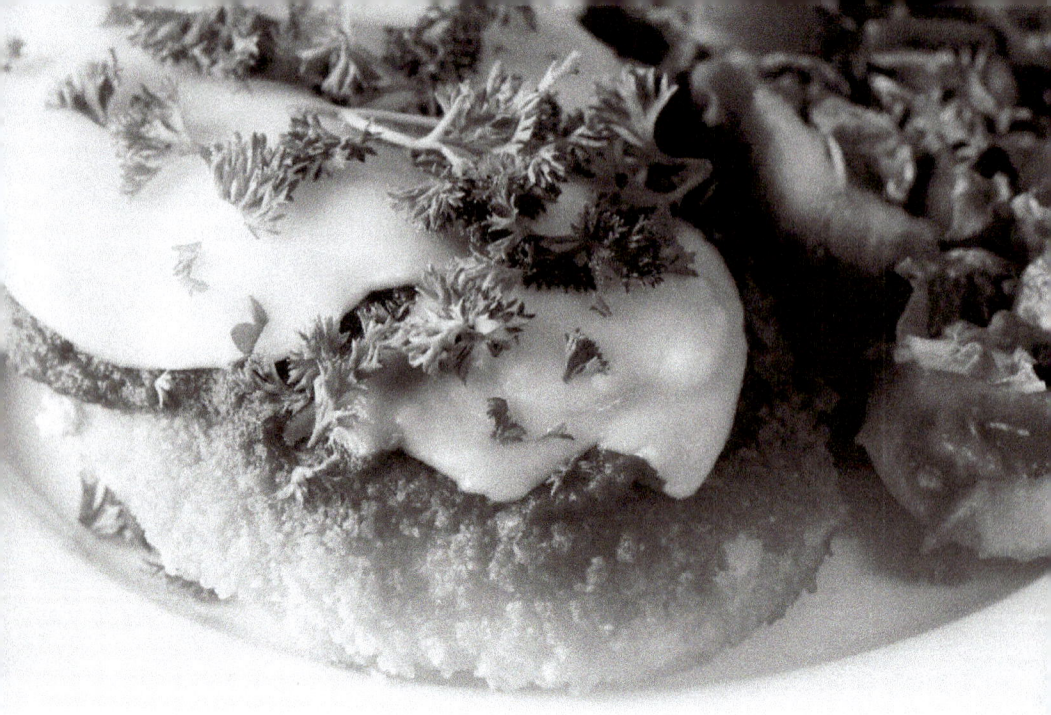

Chicken Parmesan

Serves 6

INGREDIENTS:

- 1 lb. whole wheat or gluten free linguine (try chickpea pasta). Cook pasta according to package directions
- 1 bottle marinara sauce or homemade sauce
- 3 medium boneless skinless chicken breasts, butterflied about ½ " thick to create 6 cutlets. Coat lightly with salt and pepper.
- 1 cup whole wheat or gluten free flour
- 3 eggs, beaten
- 2 cups whole wheat or gluten free breadcrumbs
- ¼ cup parmesan, plus extra for serving
- 2 teaspoons dried Italian herb blend
- ½ teaspoon garlic powder
- 1 teaspoon sea salt, more to taste
- ½ cup mozzarella cheese

PROCESS:

1. Preheat the oven to 400°F
2. Lightly oil baking sheet.
3. Prepare 3 shallow bowls placing flour in 1st, beaten eggs in 2nd, and in 3rd bowl place remaining ingredients: breadcrumbs, parmesan, herbs, and sea salt.
4. Dredge chicken in flour to absorb moisture, gently knocking off excess.
5. Dip chicken into egg coating and allow excess egg to drip off.
6. Lastly, coat both sides of chicken with breadcrumbs and place on the prepared baking sheet. Repeat the process with remaining pieces.
7. Bake in preheated oven for 15 min.
8. Remove from oven, turn breasts over and bake another 5-10 minutes, until no longer pink in center.
9. Remove from oven and top each breast with marinara sauce and shredded mozzarella.
10. Return to oven and heat until cheese is melted. Approximately 5 minutes.

Serve chicken parmesan with a side of pasta topped with marinara and sprinkle with parmesan cheese.

ACTIVITY – EMBRACE AND LOVE MOVEMENT

Housework is an often-overlooked source of physical activity that can offer significant health benefits. I tend to procrastinate when planning to clean the whole house on a Saturday. Instead, I break it up into daily tasks. I'll get up from my computer to clean a bathroom or sweep the floor while on personal phone calls. I've become the queen of cleaning multi-tasking!

Vacuum and Sweep with Purpose:

- Move briskly and add lunges or squats to your routine. By varying your movements and engaging your leg muscles, you turn a simple cleaning task into an effective lower body workout. Incorporate wide, alternating side reaches, which helps to tone your waistline.

Turn Window Cleaning into Toning:

- Reach high and low while wiping down windows, using a step stool for higher spots to maximize your stretch. This movement not only helps tone your arms and shoulders but also engages your core for a more comprehensive workout.

Laundry Workout:

- Turn laundry time into a workout by carrying heavy baskets up and down stairs or around the house to mimic weightlifting. Incorporate squats while picking up or putting down the baskets to engage your legs.

Dishwashing Dance:

- Turn dishwashing into a lively activity by swaying, stepping side to side, or even dancing as you scrub and rinse. To make this chore a delightful part of your day, play your favorite upbeat music to maintain a cheerful rhythm.

By transforming daily housework into a dynamic activity, you can maintain a clean home while staying physically fit.

KINDNESS – CULTIVATE IT IN YOUR DAILY LIFE

With the popularity of online shopping, delivery drivers work tirelessly to ensure our packages arrive on time. Surprising your delivery driver with a bag of snacks and drinks at your doorstep is an impactful way to express your gratitude and kindness.

Drinks:

- Include bottled water, flavored sparkling water and juice pouches. Vitamin Water or electrolyte drinks are especially appreciated during hot weather. Avoid energy drinks or high sugar sodas.

Healthy Snacks:

- Including items like granola bars, individual bags of mixed nuts, cheese crackers, trail mix or dried fruit sticks will offer a nutritious option for drivers who may not have time to stop for a meal.

Sweet Treats:

- Sometimes, a small, sweet treat can provide a much-needed boost to keep someone going. Consider adding individually wrapped cookies, or chocolates (when the weather is cool). These goodies can offer a moment of joy and comfort during a long workday.

Leave a Personal Note:

- Be sure to leave a clear note indicating that the bag of treats is for the delivery driver. Including a heartfelt message expressing your appreciation adds a personal touch, letting delivery drivers know their efforts are recognized and valued. This can boost their morale in a job that is often fast-paced and lonely. Consider signing the note with something personal, like "Thanks for all you do! - The Jones Family."

Surprising package delivery drivers with their own special package will brighten their day!

Log Today's Activities and Experiences with The SPEAK Method

Use the questions or comments as a guide or write freely expressing your thoughts!

SELF-CARE – When is your first "Solo Date"?

_____
_____
_____
_____
_____
_____
_____
_____

PASSION – List your "Why" questions.

_____
_____
_____
_____
_____
_____
_____
_____
_____
_____

EAT AND ENJOY NOURISHING FOOD – Liat your top 2 International favorites and how you are going to make them healthy.

_____
_____
_____
_____
_____
_____
_____
_____

ACTIVITY – Which room of the house are you going to clean first?

_____
_____
_____
_____
_____
_____
_____
_____

KINDNESS – Start small with a bag for your delivery driver, don't forget the note.

ADDITIONAL NOTES

DAILY REPORT CARD OF LIFE – How did you SPEAK today?

Grade Your Day, no D's or F's Allowed!

- **A** – Amazing
- **B** – Better than yesterday
- **C** – Challenging but working on it

DAY 22

"Do not anticipate trouble or worry about what may never happen. Keep in the sunlight."
Louisa May Alcott

SELF-CARE – PRACTICE IT DAILY

By worrying about every little thing, we stress our bodies to overproduce cortisol. While it is natural to have concerns about essential matters such as food, housing and utilities, do not let smaller, less significant worries dominate your thoughts. Also, constantly worrying about the future can rob you of enjoying the present.

Set a Worry Time:

- Rather than worrying all day about big or little things, allow yourself a scheduled "worry time." Set aside this time to think about what worries you and how to address it. Do not schedule "worry time" before meals or bed. If you start to worry at other times, just say "NO, I can only worry at my scheduled time."

Perfectionism:

- Don't worry about everything being perfect. Perfectionism can lead to burnout. Embrace the beauty of imperfection and recognize that doing your best is enough. My Virgo perfectionism creates a constant internal struggle. I have learned that letting go of perfectionism in my mind allows my heart to take over.

Minor Setbacks:

- Life is full of small obstacles that can seem significant in the moment. Instead of dwelling on minor setbacks or mistakes, view them as learning opportunities and move forward with optimism.

Uncontrollable Events:

- There is no point in worrying about things that are beyond your control. Accept that some situations are unavoidable and try to focus instead on how you respond to them.

Embrace what truly matters, and remember:
Don't worry, be happy.

PASSION – DISCOVER AND IGNITE IT

Imagine yourself at 90 years old, looking back on your life. Picture the wisdom you've gained and the experiences you've cherished. Now, consider the decisions you might regret not making. This exercise can provide remarkable insight and guide you toward aligning with your passion today.

I Could Have:

- Reflect on the opportunities that you might say, "I could have pursued my passion if I had taken that leap of faith." The key is to realize that the steps you take now can prevent these regrets later.

I Should Have:

- Think about the actions you might regret not taking. "I should have spent more time with loved ones." Prioritizing relationships and meaningful connections often become clear when viewed through the lens of a long life.

I Would Have:

- Consider the dreams that remain unfulfilled. "I would have followed my true calling if I had listened to my inner voice." Acknowledging these aspirations will motivate you to pursue what truly resonates with you and lead to a more fulfilling path.

I Didn't Because:

- Reflect on the reasons you might have held back. "I didn't take risks because I was afraid of failing." Understanding these barriers helps to overcome them, empowering you to take actions instead of letting fear dictate your choices.

By envisioning your life from the perspective of your 90-year-old self, you will gain clarity on what truly matters and guide you to make decisions that align with your passion.

EAT AND ENJOY – NOURISHING FOOD

Have you ever eaten at a restaurant and thought, "I wish I could make this dish at home"? Bon Appetit magazine used to feature a section called R.S.V.P., where readers could request recipes from their favorite restaurants. Although the magazine did not choose to publish my recipe for "Murph's Meatloaf", it was truly an honor to have this coveted recipe from my friend Murph requested by a reader. Enjoy my healthy version of **"Murph's Meatloaf".**

Ask Restaurant for Recipe:

- Chefs at local restaurants often appreciate it when you ask for their recipes, taking it as a compliment.

Search for Copycat Recipes:

- Often, you can find copycat recipes from chain restaurants on-line. Experiment with various versions until you discover the one you like best and make a healthy version.

Share with Chef Friend:

- When dining out, ask the wait staff to describe the dish, especially if it features a special sauce or seasoning. As a chef, I enjoy the challenge of recreating the recipe. If you are not a chef, snap a picture to share the dish details with your chef friends.

Watch Cooking Shows:

- Many cooking shows feature recipes from top restaurants, but one of my favorites is *Diners, Drive-Ins and Dives*. This popular Food Network show, hosted by the well-known chef Guy Fieri, takes viewers on a journey across the United States, highlighting small, often family-owned restaurants known for their unique and mouth-watering dishes.

***Gather your friends and experiment with
new recipes to make cooking a fun activity.***

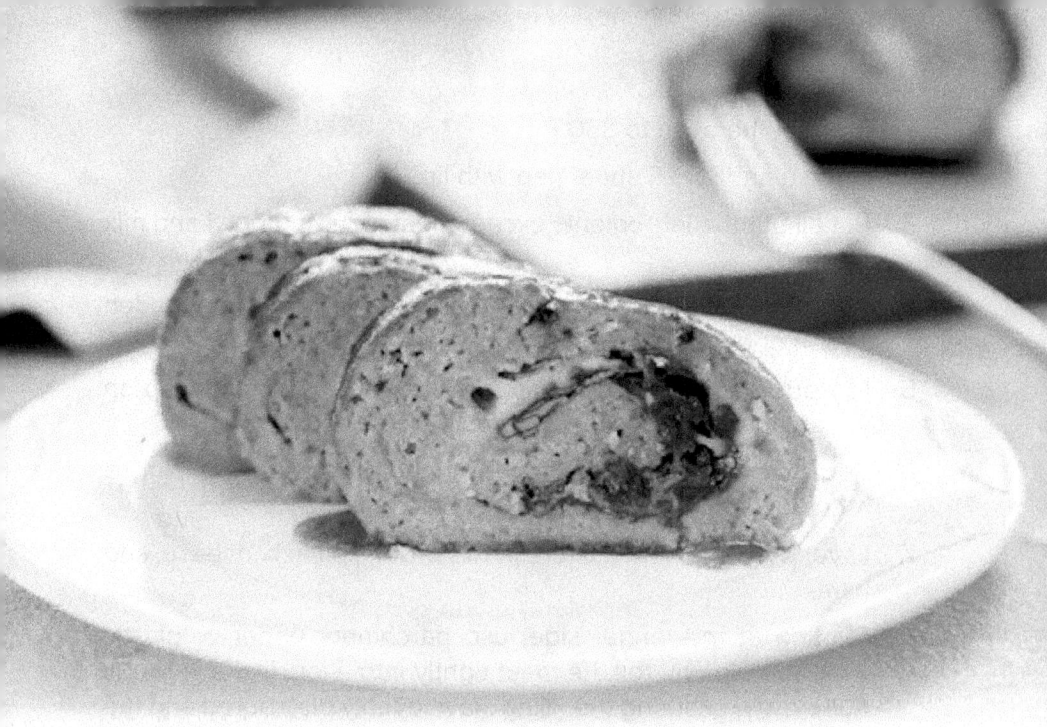

Murph's Meatloaf

6-8 Servings

INGREDIENTS:

- 1/2 cup yellow onion finely diced
- 3/4 cup raw rolled oats – not quick oats
- 1 egg, beaten
- 1/3 cup tomato juice
- 1/4 cup prepared horseradish – this is the pure stuff
- 1 teaspoon salt and pepper to taste
- 1 teaspoon dry mustard
- 2 teaspoons basil leaf
- 1 Tablespoon oregano leaf
- 1 lb. ground turkey
- 1 lb. Italian turkey sausage

For stuffing:

- 8 oz. fresh baby spinach
- 6 thin slices ham
- 6 thin slices Swiss cheese

1. Preheat the oven to 350°F
2. Grease an 18 x 26 sheet pan with lip.
3. Put all but the ingredients except meat in mixing bowl and mix well.
4. Add meat and incorporate. This is best done with a wooden spoon or even better with your hands,
5. Lay out a large piece of parchment paper or plastic wrap on your work surface.
6. Spread the meat mixture evenly on the paper, shaping it into a rectangular layer 1/2 to 3/4 inch thick.
7. Layer over the meat mixture in this order; spinach, cheese, and ham.
8. Starting at the longer side, use parchment paper or plastic wrap to help you roll the meat tightly into a log, like a jelly roll. Roll slowly, ensuring the filling stays evenly distributed and the meat rolls tightly.
9. Pinch the seam and the ends to seal the meatloaf, so the filling doesn't escape during cooking.
10. Carefully place the rolled meatloaf seam-side down on a greased baking sheet or in a loaf pan.
11. Bake 45 minutes until 165°F.
12. Top with mixture of ⅓ cup, 3 Tablespoons brown sugar and 1 Tablespoon yellow mustard and bake additional 10-15 minutes until reaches 165°F.

ACTIVITY – EMBRACE AND LOVE MOVEMENT

When it comes to incorporating daily movement, adopt the motto: "No excuses." As a health coach, I have guided individuals with arms in slings, in wheelchairs, and even a remarkable young man without any limbs. They all embraced the "No excuses" mindset and found ways to stay active.

Knee Issues:

- Swimming is an excellent full-body workout that avoids stressing the knees or ride a recumbent bicycle, adjusted to your comfort level. Having dislocated both of my knees, I am mindful to take care of them but do not use it as an excuse to be inactive.

Bad Back:

- While walking keeps you active and can be gentle on the spine, it is also important to build the core. Try pelvic tilts: Lie on your back with your knees bent and feet flat on the floor, hip-width apart, arms at sides. Exhale and engage your abdominal muscles while gently tilting your pelvis upwards and flatten your lower back against the floor.

Foot and Ankle Problems:

- Build upper body strength training with seated or standing in one place exercises, with the additional use of weights. Try resistance band workouts that focus on the upper body and core.

Neck and Shoulder Injuries:

- Practice gentle yoga, focusing on poses that stretch and strengthen the neck and shoulders without overexertion. Slow seated arm circles help improve shoulder mobility gently.

Even with injuries, there is always a safe way to keep moving and stay active. Check with your doctor to approve new movements.

KINDNESS – CULTIVATE IT IN YOUR DAILY LIFE

One powerful way to practice kindness is by making a conscious effort to remember details about the people you interact with. By paying attention and recalling these small details, you foster deeper connections. Throughout my years of health coaching, I've found this to be invaluable in forming strong client relationships.

Who to Remember:

- Practice this with everyone you interact with, from close friends and family to coworkers and even casual acquaintances. Remembering small details about people in different areas of your life signals respect and interest.

What to Remember:

- Remembering meaningful details such as favorite hobbies, important life dates, preferences (like favorite foods or colors), and any significant life events they've shared with you. These details may seem small, but they can have a big impact when brought up in future conversations.

How to Remember:

- Utilize methods such as repeating the information internally, linking the detail to something familiar, or writing down notes after your conversations. An easy approach is to add these notes to the contact section on your phone.

When to Remember:

- Bring up details about the person during subsequent interactions, whether in person or through messages. If someone told you about an upcoming event or challenge, follow up on it the next time you talk. This shows that you've been thinking about them and care about their well-being

By making a deliberate effort to remember important details about the people you interact with, you help them feel valued and appreciated.

Log Today's Activities and Experiences with The SPEAK Method

Use the questions or comments as a guide or write freely expressing your thoughts!

SELF-CARE – List things you worry about and when is your designated worry time going to be.

_____
_____
_____
_____
_____
_____

PASSION – List your "I Could Haves", "I Should Haves", "I Would Haves" and "I Didn't Because" excuses.

_____
_____
_____
_____
_____
_____
_____

EAT AND ENJOY NOURISHING FOOD – List a few your favorite restaurant dishes and try to make them at home.

_____

_____

_____

_____

_____

_____

_____

ACTIVITY – What joint issues do you have and what joint friendly exercises are you excited to try?

_____

_____

_____

_____

_____

_____

_____

KINDNESS – List two people and the details you remember about them.

_____
_____
_____
_____
_____
_____

ADDITIONAL NOTES

_____
_____
_____
_____
_____
_____

DAILY REPORT CARD OF LIFE – How did you SPEAK today?

Grade Your Day, no D's or F's Allowed!

- **A** – Amazing
- **B** – Better than yesterday
- **C** – Challenging but working on it

Interview
McKinley – Entrepreneur, Digital Marketer and Inspiration Coach

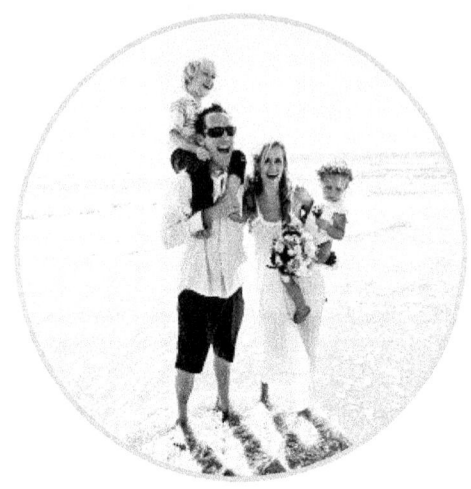

SELF-CARE – PRACTICE IT DAILY

Self-care and self-love are extremely important to me as they go hand in hand. Practicing meditation is a huge part of my life. Dr. Joe Dispenza's meditation guides have been extremely important and helpful in my journey toward unconditional self-love and forgiveness. Once I had success with these, I was able to extend the same love and forgiveness to others. One of the best things I have learned is that it starts with you first. Once you get yourself right, you can help other people.

Family and work demands are always a lot for everybody. What I find helpful is putting on a guided meditation before I go to sleep at night, there are a lot of good ones on You Tube, including Dr. Joe Dispenza's. Even with work demands, I try to find 30 minutes in the afternoon to do meditation. Some other self-care practices I do for my health and happiness include taking the right supplements, enjoying ice baths, and daily saunas.

PASSION – DISCOVER AND IGNITE IT

Passion is what drives me to find the best version of myself. If you have ever had chronic pain and figured out how to get yourself out of it, that is a very addictive feeling. So many people become addicted to feeling bad that they get used to these patterns in their lives. But once you start feeling good, it is a whole different level of passion because you don't want to go back to where you were.

What helped me ignite my passion was the feeling that I was going to lose my turn in life, and I was not going to be able to do what I loved; snowboard, skateboard, surf and do stuff with my kids. Something that has always driven me and helped me discover my passion is not wanting to lose my livelihood. Many times, I had to figure out how to get that livelihood back and it did take some passion to do that.

EAT AND ENJOY – NOURISHING FOOD

I love organic raw food, cage-free, antibiotic-free, and hormone-free foods. As Hippocrates said, "Let food be your medicine and medicine be your food." I saw what happened to my son when he was consuming too much bread. We even called him "bread boy." This led to a gluten allergy that almost caused an autoimmune disease called celiac. It was terrifying; he was sitting in class one day when his vision worsened, and his heart started palpitating. Luckily, we got blood work, and it turned out it was all because of gluten. In today's food chain, there is a lot of stuff in our food that is causing many food allergies. To have that happen at my house was a big deal. He is back to normal now, and all we had to do was cut out gluten. Having good, nourishing food is so important to my family. The other thing we did was cut out white sugar and minimize caffeine and alcohol.

ACTIVITY – EMBRACE AND LOVE MOVEMENT

One thing I do for a living is spend a significant amount of screentime on the computer. To counteract this, I prioritize getting up and moving. Using a stand-up desk has been incredibly beneficial, allowing me to work without sitting for long periods. I also make sure I take breaks every couple of hours to stretch or go for a short walk. Living near the beach, one of my favorite activities is surfing with my son and enjoying beach time with my family. It's vital to stay active because, as they say, "If you don't use it, you lose it!"

KINDNESS – CULTIVATE IT IN YOUR DAILY LIFE

Kindness is huge for me. Kathy has been an inspiration and a great teacher to me regarding kindness. When you cultivate kindness in your daily life, things change. When you really care about helping other people, that is the key to unlocking everything. The more I help people and the kinder I am to people the more of that energy I get back. I just can't put enough emphasis on the importance of kindness. The old golden rule, "Do unto others what you would want done for yourself", and maybe just a little bit more. Kindness is everything!

codymckinley@gmail.com

DAY 23

> "You can't always be worrying about what comes next. Focus on now and the little things will take care of themselves."
> **Marie Lu**

SELF-CARE – PRACTICE IT DAILY

Prioritizing is a crucial aspect of self-care. If you allow yourself to obsess over the small stuff and become overwhelmed, the important things often get pushed to the back burner. As someone who is detail oriented, I've often found myself caught up in the minutiae when working on a project, losing sight of the bigger picture. Take this book, for instance. I became overly focused on the layout instead of the main goal: sharing my heartfelt passion to help people feel younger at any age. By focusing on my passion, everything else fell into place.

Identify Your Key Goals:

- Start by clearly defining your most important personal or professional goals. Aim to focus your efforts on activities and tasks that directly support these objectives.

Utilize Tools:

- A former president created the *Eisenhower Matrix*, a task management tool that divides tasks into four quadrants to help organize and prioritize tasks based on urgency and importance.
1. Do First: Urgent and important tasks.
2. Schedule: Important but not urgent tasks.
3. Delegate: Urgent but not important tasks.
4. Delegate: Neither urgent nor important tasks.

Set Clear Deadlines:

- Assign specific deadlines to your tasks. This helps create a sense of urgency and ensures that you stay on track to complete tasks in a timely manner.

Review and Adjust Regularly:

- Regularly review your priorities and adjust as needed. Life and work circumstances change, so it's important to remain flexible.

Focus on your end goals, and the small details will naturally fall into place.

PASSION – DISCOVER AND IGNITE IT

Remember, writing has power. Try crafting letters to your future self, envisioning the passions you will be pursuing. This will help clarify what truly matters to you now. Write letters for different life stages (5, 10, 20 years from now). Ten years ago, I wrote a letter to myself about creating a cookbook, detailing the recipes, photos, and cooking tips it would include. Although this isn't purely a cookbook, it has still helped rekindle some of that passion from ten years ago.

Be Specific:
- Detail the passions you are pursuing. Instead of saying "I have created a cookbook of healthy recipes," specify "I have over 100 sugar free recipes in a cookbook, including unique and tasty desserts."

Imagine Overcoming Challenges:
- Write about obstacles you will face and how you will overcome them. For example, "Even if I encounter writer's block, I will take breaks, seek inspiration, and push through with perseverance." I will take daily walks to recharge my body and soul. "

Visualize Daily Life:
- Describe how your daily routine will look while pursuing your passions. For instance, "I will spend my mornings writing and my evenings teaching creative workshops." Describe your home, the beautiful furniture and thriving garden.

Include Personal Touches:
- Mention relationships or hobbies that support your journey. For instance, "I maintain strong connections with my female friends, meeting twice a year," and "I enjoy a week at the beach every year with my husband and my dog Mollie."

Writing letters to yourself is a powerful way to create a tangible roadmap for your journey.

EAT AND ENJOY – NOURISHING FOOD

Holidays are a special time to reunite with family and friends. These celebrations often revolve around sharing delicious meals, featuring beloved family favorites and cherished recipes that bring everyone together. Use It as a time to create healthy versions of traditional recipes.

Bake or Grill Meats:

- Whether it's a 4th of July BBQ, a Thanksgiving dinner, or any reason to celebrate, meat preparation should be simple. Last year, my friend Mike brought over his smoker and prepared a mouth-watering smoked brisket. We set up tents, and neighbors contributed side dishes and desserts. Engaging conversations ensued and future events were planned.

Reinvent Casseroles:

- At holiday events, side dishes and casseroles take center stage. From my niece Shannon's husband's famous stuffing and gravy to my stepdaughter's au gratin potatoes layered with Swiss chard, comfort foods bring us together. A couple of years ago, I reimagined the classic **Green Bean Casserole**. It quickly became a family favorite, requested every year.

Include Vegetables:

- Prepare a veggie tray with hummus and dip. Add a fun salad, such as a healthy twist on Waldorf Salad. Experiment with a new potato salad or coleslaw recipe. Roasted root vegetables make for an unexpected treat.

Enjoy Dessert:

- Include fruit-based desserts; my sister's Minnesota Apple Crisp is always a hit. Try grilling peaches for a BBQ, served with a side of ice cream, and don't forget the pumpkin pie at Thanksgiving.

These celebrations not only revolve around sharing delicious meals but also create memories that will last a lifetime.

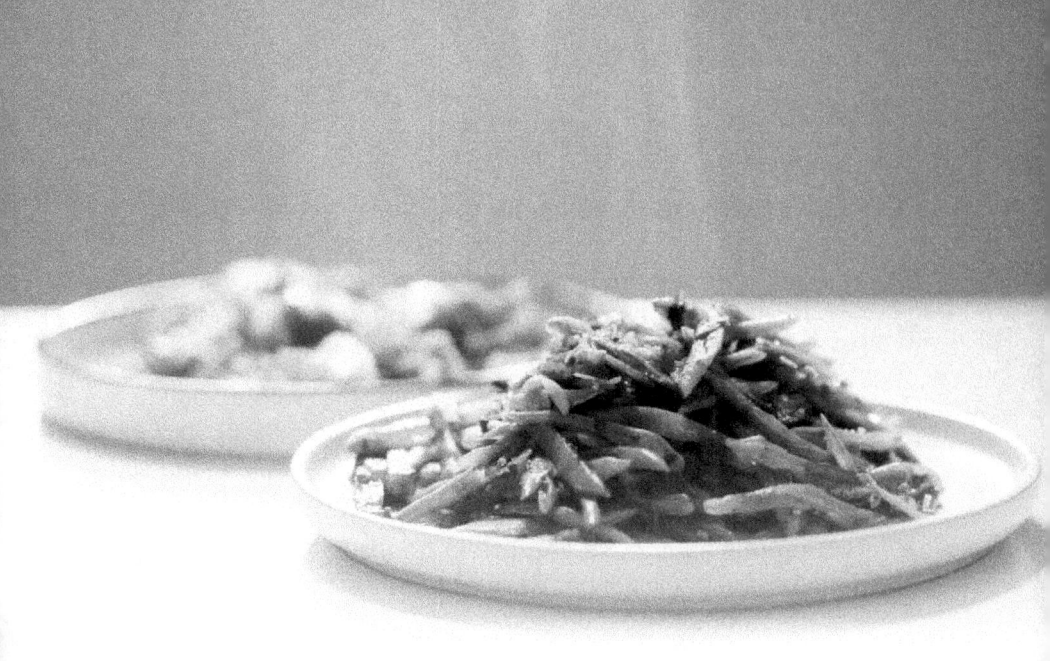

Green Bean Casserole

Serves 6

INGREDIENTS:

- 2 Tablespoons olive oil
- ½ cup mushrooms, minced
- ½ cup chopped onion
- 3 cloves garlic, minced or 1 teaspoon garlic powder
- 2 teaspoons Italian herb blend
- ¼ teaspoon smoked paprika
- ½ teaspoon sea salt
- ¼ teaspoon cracked black pepper
- 8 oz. cream cheese, softened and cut into small cubes
- 1 cup chicken or vegetable broth, no sugar added
- ¼ cup shredded parmesan cheese
- 1 16 oz. bag French cut frozen green beans, thawed or 4 cups fresh slice green beans lightly steamed and cooled
- 1 cup toasted slivered almonds or French onions topping,

PROCESS:

1. Preheat oven to 350°F
2. Place a medium saucepan on medium heat and add olive oil. When shimmering add mushrooms, onions, and garlic. Cook for 3 to 5 minutes until mushrooms begin to brown and onions are translucent, being careful not to brown garlic. Add Italian herbs, paprika, salt, and pepper, stir to combine.
3. Add cream cheese cubes to pan stirring well with a spatula to melt cream cheese. Using a whisk slowly pour stock into pan until cream cheese is melted. Turn heat down to low and simmer for 3-5 minutes or until mixture begins to thicken.
4. Add parmesan cheese and green beans to pan and mix well to combine. Pour into casserole dish and top with almonds or French onions.
5. Bake 15-20 minutes until bubbly and topping is crisp.

ACTIVITY – EMBRACE AND LOVE MOVEMENT

Group exercise transforms the nostalgia of gym classes and team selection anticipation into an organized "movement with a group." It fosters camaraderie, motivation, and a shared sense of achievement. Engaging in physical activities together not only boosts fitness but also enhances social connections.

Choose Your Sport:

- Pick a sport or activity that you enjoy, such as golf, basketball, yoga, or a baseball league. Alternatively, try the latest trending activity: pickleball, which is gaining popularity for its fun and engaging gameplay suitable for all ages. My friend Roy experienced pickleball and now teaches it to others.

Connect with a Group:

- Join a local club, class, or online community that shares your interest in the chosen sport or activity. Community centers or YMCAs often offer a variety of classes and group exercise sessions. Also, check out local Facebook groups—I discovered a women's golf lesson, a hiking group, and a beginner's pickleball group this way.

Participate in Challenges:

- Join group fitness challenges or events like charity runs or team tournaments to keep motivated. Stay informed about local events on your city's website. In my town, our Thanksgiving Turkey Trot promotes exercise before the big meal.

Mix It Up:

- Occasionally change the activity or location to keep things exciting and discover new ways to stay active with a group. Exploring different venues or trying new exercises will keep you from being bored and make your fitness routine more enjoyable.

Group exercise turns traditional gym classes of old into fun, social activities.

KINDNESS – CULTIVATE IT IN YOUR DAILY LIFE

A simple way to practice kindness is to hold back judgment and offer understanding when someone makes a mistake. Be kind to yourself as well and allow for mistakes. Often, quick judgment leads to misunderstandings and can escalate situations. A mistake is really a "miss-take," and just like in the movies, we are allowed some "re-takes."

Think Before You React:

- In the heat of the moment, we often say things we later regret. It's sometimes best to pause, take a few deep breaths, and reflect, allowing emotions to settle before responding thoughtfully and kindly. Sometimes saying, "Let's take a walk and discuss this further," immediately diffuses the situation.

Be in Their Shoes:

- Show empathy by saying, "I understand" or "I've been in that situation." This simple gesture fosters connection and reassurance, letting others know they are not alone in their experiences and feelings.

Help Find Solutions:

- View mistakes as learning opportunities. As a business owner, both I and my employees have made plenty of mistakes. Embrace these moments to grow and improve. This approach can also strengthen relationships within your family, friends or team.

Casual Follow-Up:

- Invite the person, along with others involved, to coffee or lunch. A different setting can help diffuse the situation. Encourage laughter and camaraderie to foster a positive atmosphere. Leave the door open for further positive discussions.

By practicing holding back judgment, we create a more compassionate and supportive environment for everyone.

Log Today's Activities and Experiences with The SPEAK Method

Use the questions or comments as a guide or write freely expressing your thoughts!

SELF-CARE – List things you are prioritizing.

_____
_____
_____
_____
_____
_____
_____

PASSION – How are you going to start the first letter to yourself?

_____
_____
_____
_____
_____
_____
_____
_____

EAT AND ENJOY NOURISHING FOOD – Keep a list of recipes you want to make for the next holiday celebration.

_____
_____
_____
_____
_____
_____
_____
_____

ACTIVITY – List group exercises you plan on exploring.

_____
_____
_____
_____
_____
_____
_____
_____
_____

KINDNESS – How do you usually diffuse a challenging situation and what ways are you going to try next time?

_____
_____
_____
_____
_____
_____

ADDITIONAL NOTES

_____
_____
_____
_____
_____
_____

DAILY REPORT CARD OF LIFE – How did you SPEAK today?

Grade Your Day, no D's or F's Allowed!

- **A** – Amazing
- **B** – Better than yesterday
- **C** – Challenging but working on it

DAY 24

"In the end, we only regret the chances we didn't take."
Lewis Carroll

SELF-CARE – PRACTICE IT DAILY

Create a self-care kit. It ensures that you have everything you need in one place to recharge and nurture yourself, especially during stressful times or low moments in your life. Your kit should start with something that's easy to access and has enough space for all your comforting items. It could be a decorative box, a wicker basket, or even a simple tote bag. Fill your self-care kit with items that engage your senses and make you feel good.

Things That Feel Good:

- Include a warm blanket to wrap yourself in for instant comfort and a soft, plush pillow to rest your head on. Add cozy slippers or socks to make you feel pampered. Finish with a stress ball to squeeze or play with when you need to release tension.

Things That Smell Good:

- Include scented candles with calming scents like lavender, vanilla, or eucalyptus. Add essential oils for therapeutic aromatherapy to help relax and uplift your mood. You might also consider including a fragrant sachet filled with dried herbs or flowers to keep your space smelling fresh.

Things that Taste Good:

- Include some healthy and indulgent snacks like dark chocolate, nuts, crackers or even a comforting soup mix. My personal favorite is miso packets as they remind me of the tasty soup served in Japanese restaurants. Add sachets of hot cocoa, herbal tea bags, or instant coffee for a quick pick-me-up.

Easily prioritize your self-care with your kit close at hand.

PASSION – DISCOVER AND IGNITE IT

The idea of creating a "pros and cons" list to help with decision-making is often attributed to Benjamin Franklin. He referred to this method as "moral algebra" or "prudential algebra". In 1772, Franklin described how he would draw a line down the middle of a piece of paper, writing the Pros on one side and the Cons on the other. He would then weigh the importance of each point until he arrived at a decision. I've used a "pro and con" list to decide on moving to Panama and even writing this book! It's incredibly helpful for many important decisions, including pursuing your passion. Here are a couple of examples of a "pros and cons" list.

Starting a New Project:

Evaluate the benefits and potential drawbacks when starting something new.

Pros:

- Brings you in contact with like-minded individuals.
- Boosts your enthusiasm and creativity.

Cons:

- May require a significant time investment.
- There is a risk that the project may not succeed as planned.

Investing in Training or Courses About Your Passion:

Weigh the investment of time and money against the skills gained.

Pros:

- Gain advanced skills and knowledge that can elevate your expertise.
- Boosts your credibility and professional reputation.

Cons:

- Training or courses can be expensive.
- Courses often require a significant time commitment.

Creating these lists will provide clarity and confidence when pursuing your passion.

EAT AND ENJOY – NOURISHING FOOD

We all know the feeling—it's mid-afternoon, and suddenly, you have an intense craving for something crispy and salty. Many times, our immediate reaction is to reach for potato chips and dips which, while tasty, aren't always the healthiest choice. Instead of succumbing to less nutritious options, consider these wholesome snack alternatives.

Spinach and Artichoke Dip:

- Make a lightened-up version with Greek yogurt, low-fat cream cheese, spinach, artichokes, garlic, Parmesan cheese, salt, and pepper. It is a tasty dip for whole-grain baguette slices, bell pepper slices, and cucumber rounds.

Greek Yogurt Tzatziki:

- A simple dip made with Greek yogurt, cucumber, garlic, lemon juice, dill, olive oil, salt, and pepper. Tzatziki is great for dipping cucumber slices, carrot or celery sticks, cherry tomatoes, snap peas and whole-grain pita chips.

Chips, Salsa and Queso:

- Skip the Mexican restaurant and make your own. Most store-bought salsas, particularly those in the Hispanic section, are made with tomatoes, peppers, onions, and spices. You could also try making a fresh Pico de Gallo or my favorite **Queso Dip** recipe. Pair it with corn chips, whole grain chips, or jicama for dipping.

Bean Dips:

- Get a burst of protein with hummus and veggies or whole-grain pita chips. Make your own refried beans by mashing canned, rinsed pintos with garlic and salsa. Melt a little cheddar cheese on top and enjoy with your corn or whole grain chips. Or turn it into a delicious plate of nachos.

Expand your salty snack choices and never feel deprived.

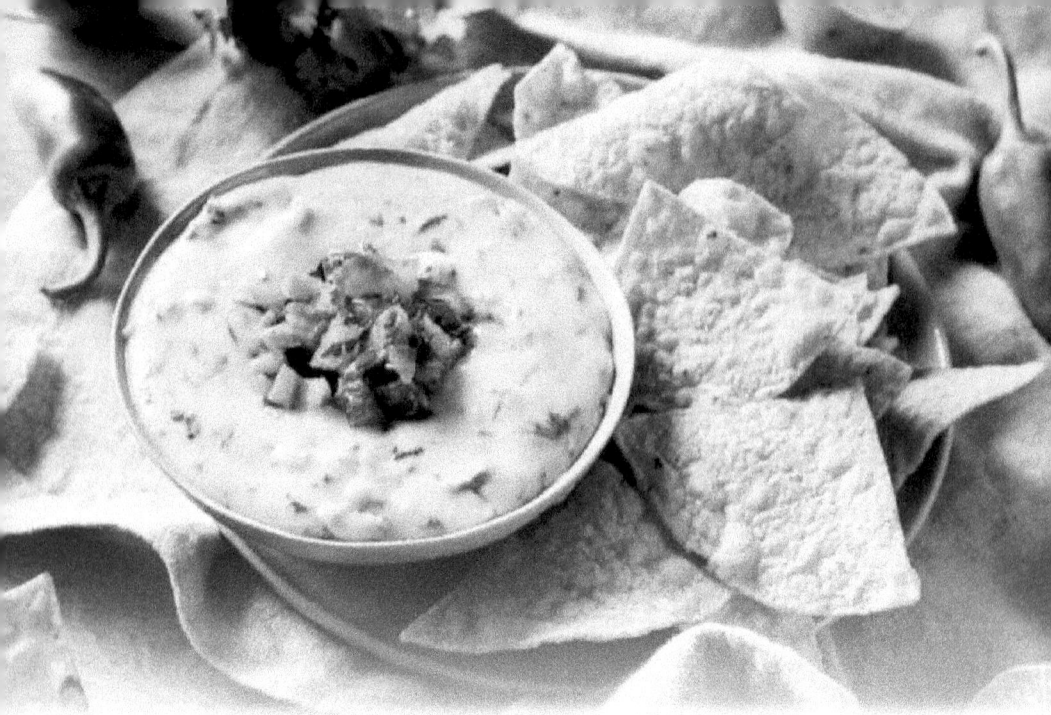

Queso Dip

8- 10 Servings

INGREDIENTS:

- 1 cup whole milk
- 3 Tablespoons cornstarch
- 1 teaspoon olive or avocado oil
- ¼ cup yellow onion, minced
- 2 garlic cloves, minced
- 1 poblano pepper (or red pepper), diced
- 1 jalapeño, seeded and diced, optional
- ½ cup chicken broth
- 1 10 oz can diced tomatoes with chiles, drained
- ¼ cup fresh cilantro, chopped 1 lime, juiced
- Sea salt, to taste
- ½ teaspoon ground cumin
- 1 teaspoon chipotle chili powder
- 1 ¾ cups shredded cheddar cheese

PROCESS:

1. In a small bowl whisk ¼ cup of the milk with cornstarch until combined and set aside.
2. Heat a large saucepan on medium heat. Add oil, onions, garlic, poblano, and jalapeno to pan cooking for 5-7 minutes until soft.
3. Season with salt, to taste. Add the chicken broth and the rest of the milk.
4. Bring to a full boil and reduce heat to medium low, simmering for 5 minutes to reduce liquid.
5. Add the milk and starch mixture to the pan and whisk to combine. Continue to simmer until it bubbles and thickens.
6. Reduce heat to low. Stir in the drained tomatoes, cilantro, lime juice, chili powder, cumin, and sea salt.
7. Remove from heat and add the cheese stirring until completely melted and serve while still warm with corn chips or wholegrain chips.

ACTIVITY – EMBRACE AND LOVE MOVEMENT

A unique and enjoyable form of exercise I tried several years ago is Bokwa, a dance fitness program that combines cardio workouts with elements of African dance and aerobics. It's a fun way to stay fit and improve balance with easy steps, making it perfect for people of all ages and fitness levels.

Basics of Bokwa:

- In Bokwa, you "write" letters and numbers with your feet while moving to upbeat music. Unlike traditional aerobics or dance classes, it doesn't require counting steps or dancing in unison.

Beginning Steps:

- Start by drawing an "L" with your feet. Step forward with your right foot, then step to the left with your left foot, creating an "L" shape on the floor.
- Create a "J" shape by stepping to the left with your left foot, then curving your right foot back to the right, like you're drawing a "J."
- For the number "1," step forward with your right foot and then back to your starting position.
- Move in the shape of a "3" by stepping forward and to the left, then curving your step back and to the right, like drawing the number "3" with your feet.
- Try all the alphabet and numbers.

Combine the Moves:

- As you become more comfortable with the steps, combine them into sequences or words.
- Create a fun Bokwa party game by seeing who "spells" a word with their feet first.

Lace up your shoes, crank up the music, and enjoy the rhythm!

KINDNESS – CULTIVATE IT IN YOUR DAILY LIFE

Showing kindness while driving is crucial for ensuring a safer and more pleasant experience for all road users. This in the car kindness can significantly reduce stress, prevent accidents, and promote a sense of community.

In Traffic:

- Traffic jams can be incredibly frustrating, but a little kindness goes a long way. Allowing other drivers to merge in front of you can ease the flow of traffic and reduce road rage. A simple wave of thanks when someone lets you in can brighten their day.

In Parking Lots:

- Parking lots can be chaotic, especially during busy hours. If you see someone waiting for a spot, be respectful and let them in. Also, be considerate of pedestrians, giving them the right of way. I was recently in a congested tourist area in Savannah, GA, and was pleasantly surprised by the kindness of the drivers—Southern hospitality at its finest.

In Downtown Walking Areas:

- Downtown areas often have heavy pedestrian traffic, so it's important to remain cautious and courteous. Yield to pedestrians at crosswalks and avoid honking unnecessarily. When parking, ensure your vehicle is entirely within the lines to avoid inconveniencing others.

In Residential Areas:

- Neighborhood driving requires extra care and consideration. Drive slowly and watch out for children playing or pets that may dart into the street. Being courteous to cyclists and giving them ample space is also important. Avoid loud music and excessive honking.

Have more fun on the road by practicing these simple acts of kindness.

Log Today's Activities and Experiences with The SPEAK Method

Use the questions or comments as a guide or write freely expressing your thoughts!

SELF-CARE – What are you putting in your self-care kit?

_____
_____
_____
_____
_____
_____
_____
_____

PASSION – Start your first Pro-Con List for a new passion.

_____
_____
_____
_____
_____
_____
_____
_____
_____
_____

EAT AND ENJOY NOURISHING FOOD – List your favorite salty and crispy snacks to make healthy.

_____
_____
_____
_____
_____
_____
_____
_____
_____
_____

ACTIVITY – Which letters and numbers did you draw with your feet?

_____
_____
_____
_____
_____
_____
_____
_____
_____
_____

KINDNESS – In which area of driving do you get frustrated and now plan on practicing kindness?

_____
_____
_____
_____
_____

ADDITIONAL NOTES

_____
_____
_____
_____
_____
_____

DAILY REPORT CARD OF LIFE – How did you SPEAK today?

Grade Your Day, no D's or F's Allowed!

- **A** – Amazing
- **B** – Better than yesterday
- **C** – Challenging but working on it

DAY 25

> "Cooking is like love. It should be entered into with abandon or not at all."
> **Harriet Van Horne**

SELF-CARE – PRACTICE IT DAILY

Creating a Personal Victory Log is a powerful self-care practice that helps you recognize and celebrate your achievements, no matter how small. By consistently acknowledging your successes, you can build self-worth, resilience, and a positive mindset.

Choose Your Journal:

- Choose a journal or notebook specifically for your Personal Victory Log. It can be a simple notebook, a journal in your favorite color, or even a digital app if you prefer typing. Alternatively, you can use the "Additional Notes" section in this book at the end of each day to record your victories. The key is to select something that feels comfortable and accessible to you.

Acknowledge All Wins:

- Victories don't have to be grand; they can be as simple as getting out of bed on a challenging day, completing a task, taking a walk, or setting aside time for yourself. No matter the size, every accomplishment matters.

Categories of Victories:

- Consider thinking about different categories of achievements, like personal growth, work-related successes, or health and wellness victories. This helps recognize achievements across your life. For example, I record my movement victories weekly, noting specifics like walking, lifting weights , and dancing at a concert.

Use It as a Tool for Resilience

- When you're feeling down or facing challenges, go back to your Victory Log and read through your past achievements. This can remind you of your strengths and capabilities, boosting your confidence to overcome obstacles.

Recall the quote from the movie, "The Help":
"You is kind. You is smart. You is important."

PASSION – DISCOVER AND IGNITE IT

Create a Legacy Project: Undertake a mission that you want to be remembered for—be it writing a book, creating art, or initiating a community project. Concentrating on what you wish to leave behind can uncover your deeper purpose. My legacy project involves coaching people to feel youthful at any age, and I plan to continue doing so well into my 90s, and possibly even 100!

Create a Lasting Impact:

- Focus on passions that will have a long-term impact. Making a lasting impact means thinking big and aiming for sustainable change that will leave a legacy for future generations.

Set Clear Goals:

- Outline specific, measurable, achievable, relevant, and time-frame goals for your project. Clear goals will guide your efforts and keep you focused. As a procrastinator, I set a specific goal with a deadline to finish this writing project. Be careful not to overcommit and set yourself up for disappointment.

Engage Others:

- Involve friends, family or like-minded individuals in your project. Collaboration not only enriches your legacy but also ensures sustainability and a wider impact. Even the "Lone Ranger," a TV show from the 1950s, had his trusted companion Tonto as he rode into the sunset shouting, "Hi-Ho Silver, Away!"

Seek Continuous Improvement:

- Regularly review and refine your project to stay relevant and effective. Gather feedback, stay updated with trends, and embrace new ideas to ensure continuous improvement, fostering growth and maximizing its long-term impact.

Just like mine, your Legacy Project will evolve over time.

EAT AND ENJOY – NOURISHING FOOD

Fat-free diets gained popularity in the 1970s and 1980s due to research linking high-fat diets to heart disease and other chronic conditions. Unfortunately, the difference between good and bad fats was overlooked. My mom used butter until advertisers convinced her to switch to Oleo margarine. Margarines are highly processed, contain trans fats, and have higher Omega-6 fatty acids, contributing to inflammation. Choose healthy oils instead.

Olive Oil:

- A heart-healthy choice that improves blood pressure, cholesterol, and reduces inflammation. Ideal for salad dressings, marinades, and low-temp sautéing. Avoid high heat; it turns unhealthy when it smokes. Enjoy the **Three Citrus Vinaigrette** in salads and marinades.

Avocados and Avocado Oil:

- Packed with healthy fats, fiber, vitamins, and antioxidants, they promote heart health, improve digestion, and support skin vitality. Avocado oil, rich in monounsaturated fats, is perfect for high heat cooking due to its high smoke point.

Coconut Oil:

- Coconut oil: Rich in medium-chain triglycerides (MCTs) that boost energy and metabolism. Enhances skin and hair health; usable both internally and externally. Ideal for cooking, baking, and smoothies. With a high smoke point, it's suitable for sautéing and frying. I kickstart my day with a teaspoon of coconut oil in my morning coffee.

Butter:

- Butter not only enriches flavor but also provides essential vitamins A, D, E, and K, promotes healthy skin, and supports brain function. Choose grass-fed options, Irish butter or local artisanal butters for optimal benefits.

Enjoy these healthy fats while also benefiting from their ability to keep you full.

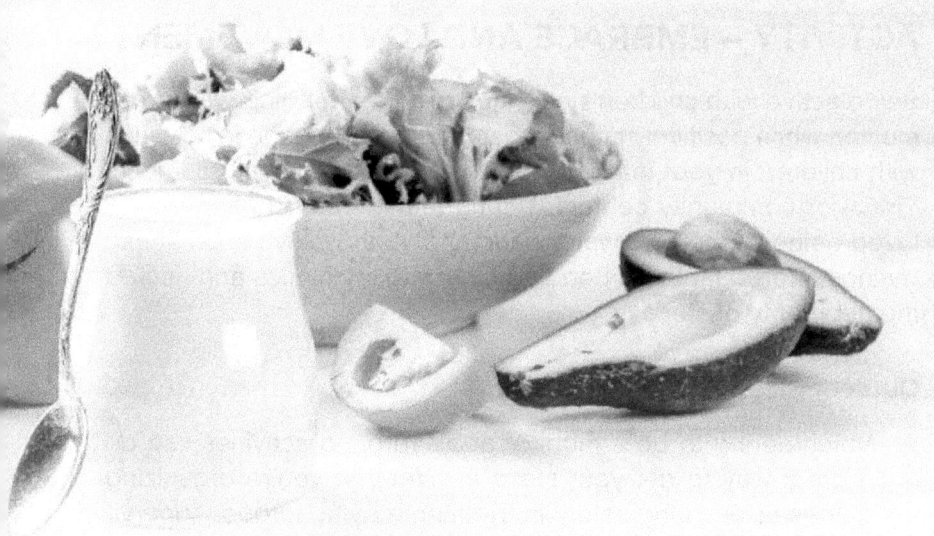

Three Citrus Vinaigrette

Makes 1 Heaping Cup

INGREDIENTS:

- ¼ cup apple cider vinegar
- 2 Tablespoons fresh orange juice
- 2 Tablespoons fresh lemon juice
- ¾ cup olive oil
- 1 teaspoon lime zest
- 1 teaspoon orange zest
- 1 teaspoon lemon zest
- 1 Tablespoon honey
- ¼ teaspoon salt
- ¼ teaspoon fresh ground black pepper optional

PROCESS:

1. Combine all vinaigrette ingredients except for olive oil to a small mixing bowl and whisk well.
2. While continuing to whisk, add olive oil in a slow, steady stream until fully incorporated.
3. Alternately, put all ingredients in glass jar and shake well.
4. Drizzle vinaigrette on top of salad or coleslaw or use as a marinade for chicken, fish or pork.

ACTIVITY – EMBRACE AND LOVE MOVEMENT

Being active with children's activities can be a fulfilling way to get moving while positively impacting young lives. Engage in activities with children in your family or look for opportunities at your local YMCA or community centers. During family visits in Minnesota, I loved going to the zoo, water park, and various city parks. These outings offered fantastic bonding time with my nieces and helped me get plenty of steps in.

Outdoor Play:

- Volunteering to be a monitor at playground activities can be a great way to get your steps in. Whether you're organizing games or ensuring safety in the jungle gym, outdoor supervision keeps you active and engaged.

Sports or Dance Clinics:

- Offering your expertise in sports, such as soccer, basketball, swimming or dance classes, keeps you physically active while teaching children valuable skills. It also encourages them to stay fit and develop a love for physical activity. No experience needed—many classes or clinics are looking for helpers.

Group Games:

- Leading or assisting in group games like baseball, relay races, tennis or sport of your choice not only gets your heart pumping but also teaches kids about teamwork and fair play. It's a fun way to incorporate cardio into your routine.

Nature Walks:

- Lead or assist in educational nature walks. This activity combines movement with learning, as you explore local parks or trails, teaching children about various plants and animals they encounter.

Always remember, one of the most important things is to laugh and have fun!

KINDNESS – CULTIVATE IT IN YOUR DAILY LIFE

An easy yet impactful act of kindness is jotting down uplifting messages on pieces of paper or sticky notes and leaving them in public places. This modest act has the potential to brighten someone's day and serve as a reminder that kindness is everywhere.

Where to Put Notes:

- Choose places where people are likely to notice the notes but won't be bothered by them. Mirrors in restrooms, public transportation seats, communal bulletin boards, and inside library books are excellent options. These spots ensure your positive messages will be seen by many and can offer a quick boost of joy.

What to Write:

- Keep your messages simple, heartfelt, and uplifting. Phrases like "You are amazing!", "Believe in yourself!", or "You have the power to make a difference!" work wonderfully. Make sure your words are encouraging and can resonate with a wide audience.

Use Bright Colors:

- Eye-catching colors such as yellow, pink, or orange are more likely to grab attention. A bright, cheerful sticky note can stand out even in a crowded or busy area, making sure your message is noticed.

Add Little Drawings:

Including a small doodle can often enhance your message. When possible, involve children by asking them to draw hearts, small flowers, or smiley faces on the notes. This adds a personal touch and makes the note feel more special and intentional.

Leaving positive notes is a small act that can have a big positive impact!

Log Today's Activities and Experiences with The SPEAK Method

Use the questions or comments as a guide or write freely expressing your thoughts!

SELF-CARE – List the first entries for your Personal Victory Log.

_____
_____
_____
_____
_____
_____
_____
_____

PASSION – Write some of the Legacies you are exploring.

_____
_____
_____
_____
_____
_____
_____
_____

EAT AND ENJOY NOURISHING FOOD – How do you currently use healthy fats? Ideas for expanding your recipes to include them?

_____
_____
_____
_____
_____
_____
_____
_____
_____

ACTIVITY – What children do you love to play with? List new movement activities to play with them?

_____
_____
_____
_____
_____
_____
_____
_____
_____

KINDNESS – Get out your sticky notes or small pieces of paper and start writing positive messages. Put in your car or purse. Where will your first post be?

_____
_____
_____
_____
_____
_____

ADDITIONAL NOTES

_____
_____
_____
_____
_____
_____
_____

DAILY REPORT CARD OF LIFE – How did you SPEAK today?

Grade Your Day, no D's or F's Allowed!

- **A** – Amazing
- **B** – Better than yesterday
- **C** – Challenging but working on it

DAY 26

"Dessert is like a feel-good song and the best ones make you dance."
Chef Edward Lee

SELF-CARE – PRACTICE IT DAILY

Dedicate time to reading for self-care. Choose books that inspire you, bring joy, or allow you to escape to another world. This practice nurtures your mind, reduces stress, and fosters a sense of relaxation and happiness. Choose a quiet, comfortable spot, grab a blanket and a cup of tea. While paper books are ideal, eBooks or audiobooks are also convenient options.

Mystery Novels:

- These books offer suspense, mental engagement, and excitement, allowing us to solve puzzles, escape reality, and enjoy thrilling plots.

Fantasy Books:

- This genre of books ignites imagination, transports readers to magical worlds, and inspires creativity while offering thrilling adventures and escape from reality. My all-time favorite is J.R.R Tolkien's "The Hobbit" and "Lord of the Rings".

Science Fiction:

- These books spark imagination and expand your horizons. They allow you to explore the potential impact of new technology and offer thrilling adventures beyond reality. One of the first scary science fiction books I read was "The Time Machine" by H.G. Wells.

Romance Novels:

- Providing emotional escape, inspiring hope, and offering valuable insights into relationships, these books can enhance your empathy and imagination. My sweet younger sister Anne was an avid reader of Danielle Steele, the steamier the better.

Historical Fiction:

- Immerse yourself in past eras that offer insights into historical events. These books bring history to life and foster a deeper understanding of different cultures.

Escape to another world within your favorite book.

PASSION – DISCOVER AND IGNITE IT

Free writing is an uninhibited writing exercise where you write continuously for a set period without worrying about grammar, spelling, or topic coherence. The aim is to unlock creativity and encourage the flow of ideas. It can reveal thoughts and feelings about passions you never knew existed. I first experienced this enlightening exercise in a non-fiction writing class at the local community college, and it transformed my approach to self-expression.

Set a Time Limit:

- Choose a short time frame, typically 5-10 minutes, to write without interruptions. This approach encourages a concentrated burst of creativity, helping you focus on the flow of your ideas without the pressure of perfecting them.

Write Continuously:

- Select a comfortable pen that fits well in your hand and has plenty of ink. Keep the pen moving or fingers typing, even if you end up writing "I don't know what to write" repeatedly. This practice helps bypass mental blocks, allowing thoughts to flow freely and sparking creativity.

No Editing:

- Avoid correcting mistakes or stopping to review what you're writing. Embrace any errors without worrying about grammar or punctuation, as this promotes unrestricted creativity and helps you connect more deeply with your inner thoughts and feelings.

Focus on Flow:

- Allow your thoughts to move freely from one idea to the next without restriction. This unfiltered movement fosters greater creativity and reveals hidden insights, enabling you to explore your thoughts and emotions more deeply.

Be in a quiet space with no distractions and start writing.

EAT AND ENJOY – NOURISHING FOOD

Stressed spelled backward is desserts. Coincidence? I think not. Enjoying dessert can be guilt-free and satisfy your sweet tooth without compromising your health. By choosing treats made with natural sweeteners, fruits, and whole ingredients, you can indulge in the pleasure of desserts without feeling guilty. So, go ahead and enjoy your desserts – it's the sweetest way to de-stress!

Incorporate Fruit:

- Try honey-sweetened fresh fruit crisp with pecan oatmeal topping, fresh fruit pops, grilled pineapple or peaches with frozen yogurt, and apple cinnamon compote.

Natural Sweeteners:

- Match your sweetener's flavor with your recipe: Use honey in fruit-based desserts, maple syrup for a caramel-like flavor, monk fruit as a white sugar replacement in baking, and coconut sugar for brown sugar substitutes.

Whole Grains:

- Opt for whole wheat flour or gluten-free blends. My top choice for replacing white flour in baking is white whole wheat flour. Made from spring wheat, it is less grainy than traditional whole wheat flour and offers the light texture of white flour with the benefits of whole grains.

Nuts and Seeds:

- Enhance the nutrition of desserts with nuts and seeds, rich in healthy fats and protein. Use ground nuts or seeds to create unique pie or tart crusts and sprinkle them over ice cream or yogurt. Add nuts or seeds to your favorite muffins, cakes, cookies, and bread. For a quick sweet treat, try **Four Ingredient Peanut Butter Cookies.**

Keep calm and eat dessert, just don't overeat!

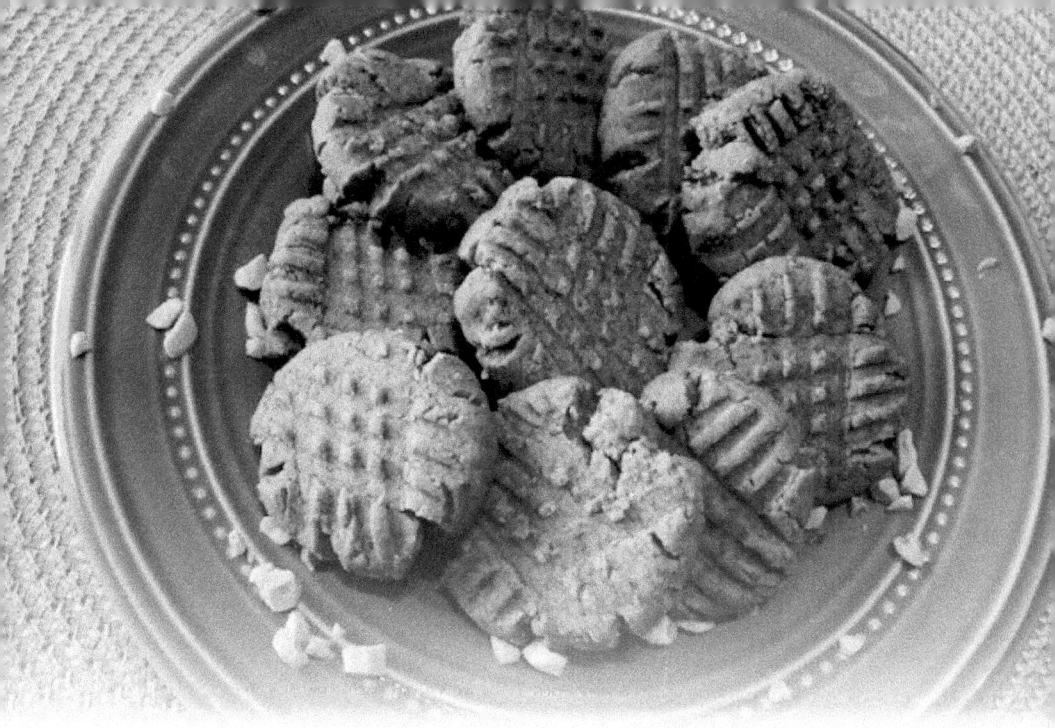

Four Ingredient Peanut Butter Cookies

14-16 Cookies

INGREDIENTS:

- 1 cup creamy sugar free peanut butter
- ½ cup coconut sugar
- ½ cup almond flour
- 1 egg

PROCESS:

1. Preheat oven to 350F.
2. Line a baking sheet with parchment paper.
3. In a medium bowl, add peanut butter and coconut sugar.
4. With a hand mixer, cream until smooth and fluffy.
5. Add egg and cream again with hand mixer.
6. While beating, add 2 Tablespoons of flour at a time until incorporated.

7. Check after adding all but the last 2 Tablespoons to see if dough forms into a ball.
8. The amount of flour will depend upon your peanut butter consistency.
9. Form into 1 inch ball and place on lined cooking sheet.
10. Use a fork to press down twice in a crisscross pattern.
11. Bake in preheated oven for 12-14 minutes until edges are slightly browned.
12. Cool on baking sheet for 2 minutes, then transfer to cooling rack.
13. After cooling, store in covered container.
14. These are also great frozen.

ACTIVITY – EMBRACE AND LOVE MOVEMENT

Relive your childhood with nostalgic games. Growing up in the '50s, long before the advent of video games, we played outdoors with our neighbors. Outdoor games boost your fitness level and evoke memories of simpler times. Gather your friends and family for laughter and fun while playing timeless games.

Blind Man's Bluff:

- One player wears a blindfold and tries to tag the others using only their sense of sound and touch. This game encourages creativity, involves plenty of circling around to find participants, and generates a lot of laughter. Play on a level, soft grassy area.

Tug of War:

- Two teams pull on opposite ends of a rope, aiming to drag the other team across a marked line. It encourages teamwork and strategic thinking while building muscle strength and endurance. Play in a flat, grassy area with plenty of open space.

Red Rover:

- Players are divided into two teams, holding hands in a line. One team calls a player from the other to run and break through their clasped hands. It builds teamwork and strengthens arms and legs. I can still hear the song: "Red rover, red rover, send somebody over."

Duck, Duck, Goose:

- Players sit in a circle. One walks around tapping heads, saying "duck" each time, until choosing a "goose" who must chase them around the circle. This game enhances reaction time with quick movements, making it perfect for all ages. Somehow, I was always picked as the goose!

Activity and laughter erase stress and anxiety!

KINDNESS – CULTIVATE IT IN YOUR DAILY LIFE

Most people are naturally kind; often, it just takes a simple conversation to bring out their warmth. Initiating a dialogue can ignite a flow of kindness, fostering connections and goodwill in your community. Small steps can lead to meaningful bonds. There are endless opportunities to strike up conversations. You never know the outcome until you try.

Volunteer Events:

- Participating in local community service or charity events is a great way to meet like-minded individuals. Starting a conversation here could lead to collaborative acts of kindness.

Shopping:

- You never know where a conversation with a store worker will lead. Before my brother-in-law's funeral, his daughter was shopping for something to wear while giving the eulogy. In the nicest store in town, a salesclerk helped her find a green blouse, as everyone was wearing green to honor Mike's Irish heritage. During their chat, the clerk mentioned she was a singer. Before leaving, the clerk offered to sing the Irish tune "Danny Boy" at the funeral, an unexpected and caring act of kindness.

Fitness Classes:

- Engaging with fellow participants in fitness classes or at the gym can build a sense of camaraderie, resulting in encouraging words and mutual support that boosts everyone's morale.

Local Markets:

- Farmers' markets or craft fairs provide a casual environment to connect with vendors and shoppers alike, often leading to kind gestures like sharing recipe tips or supporting small businesses.

Spark up conversations,
it could lead you to the kindest people!

Log Today's Activities and Experiences with The SPEAK Method

Use the questions or comments as a guide or write freely expressing your thoughts!

SELF-CARE – List books for your reading list.

_____
_____
_____
_____
_____
_____
_____
_____

PASSION – Start your free writing here.

_____
_____
_____
_____
_____
_____
_____
_____
_____

EAT AND ENJOY NOURISHING FOOD — What are your favorite desserts? How will you make them healthier?

_____
_____
_____
_____
_____
_____
_____
_____

ACTIVITY — List your favorite childhood games and who you plan on inviting to play.

_____
_____
_____
_____
_____
_____
_____
_____

KINDNESS – How are you going to initiate a conversation today?

_____
_____
_____
_____
_____
_____

ADDITIONAL NOTES

_____
_____
_____
_____
_____
_____
_____

DAILY REPORT CARD OF LIFE – How did you SPEAK today?

Grade Your Day, no D's or F's Allowed!

- **A** – Amazing
- **B** – Better than yesterday
- **C** – Challenging but working on it

DAY 27

"I spent my life accumulating wealth and then had to spend my wealth to regain my health"
Popular Proverb, Author Unknown

SELF-CARE – PRACTICE IT DAILY

Financial self-care is crucial for a balanced life, empowering you to manage your resources wisely without sacrificing your well-being. Making financial health a priority ensures stability and peace of mind, enabling you to invest in your overall well-being.

Create a Budget:

- Track your income and expenses to get a clear picture of your financial situation. A well-planned budget helps you prioritize essential spending, ensuring that your needs are met first.

Save for a Rainy Day:

- Create an emergency fund to handle unforeseen expenses or financial difficulties. Strive to save enough to cover three to six months' worth of living costs.

  Growing up in a modest family, we had our needs met but had little extra money. However, my dad always joked that he "never spent a dime." Each night, he would separate the dimes from his pocket change and put them in a special jar. That jar became our "splurge" fund. The most memorable splurge funded by those dimes was a trip to the Wisconsin Dells in the neighboring state. Get a piggy bank and start your "splurge" fund.

Invest Wisely:

- Grow your wealth by investing in diversified assets. Research and consider consulting a financial advisor to make informed decisions that align with your goals.

Reduce Debt:

- Focus on paying off high-interest debts first. Developing a strategy to manage and reduce debt can improve financial stability and reduce stress.

Live by the motto:
"Money makes good people better and bad people worse."

PASSION – DISCOVER AND IGNITE IT

As you may have noticed with The SPEAK Method, I love using acronyms. They simplify remembering important concepts. When pursuing your passion, apply the SMART acronym: Specific, Measurable, Achievable, Relevant, and Time-bound. This framework helps set clear and attainable goals.

Specific:

- When identifying what makes an activity meaningful to you, be clear and specific. Design targeted activities to explore and document those that excite you.

Measurable:

- Ensure the journey towards achieving your passion is measurable. Establish clear, attainable goals with specific milestones to assess your growth. Frequently review your journal to track your progress.

Achievable:

- To truly ignite your passion, it's crucial to set realistic and attainable goals. By breaking down your passion into manageable steps, you make the journey less overwhelming, more achievable, and increase your chances of long-term success. Never having written a book before, I initially set an unrealistic goal. Once I adjusted to a more realistic target, the thoughts and words began to flow effortlessly.

Relevant:

- Your passion should align with your broader objectives. For me, it's about helping people feel youthful at any age.

Time-bound:

- Your passion goal should have a specific deadline or a clear time frame within which it should be accomplished. This helps maintain focus and ensures steady progress towards achieving your desired outcome.

By being SMART, you will have a clearer path to discovering and igniting your passion.

EAT AND ENJOY – NOURISHING FOOD

Did you know that over 70% of your immune system resides in your gut? Often referred to as the "second brain," your gut health plays a crucial role in overall well-being. Maintaining a healthy gut can boost immunity, enhance mood, and improve digestion. Incorporate gut-healthy foods into your daily diet.

Raw Veggies:

- Raw vegetables are rich in natural enzymes that aid in the digestion and absorption of nutrients. My husband finds it unusual, but I follow the European tradition of eating salad at the end of the meal to aid in digesting the cooked dishes.

Herbs and Spices:

- Mother Nature's original medicine can be incorporated into your meals to promote better digestion.
- Ginger: Put in Asian meals or tea to alleviate nausea and stimulate digestion.
- Peppermint: Infuse water with peppermint leaves or make tea to soothe the stomach.
- Fennel: Roast or put in a salad to ease digestive issues such as bloating, gas, and constipation.
- Cumin: Great in Mexican dishes to help stimulate the secretion of digestive enzymes. Enjoy tailgate favorite, **White Chicken Chili.**

High Fiber Nuts and Seeds:

- Choose the highest fiber nuts, including almonds, pistachios, hazelnuts, and pecans. Make a pudding with chia seeds, one of the highest fiber foods. Add flaxseeds to smoothies and baked goods. Sprinkle sunflower seeds, pumpkin seeds, sesame seeds, or hemp seeds on your salad.

Also, **incorporate the fermented foods we discussed on Day 10.**

Follow the motto: Happy gut, happy life!

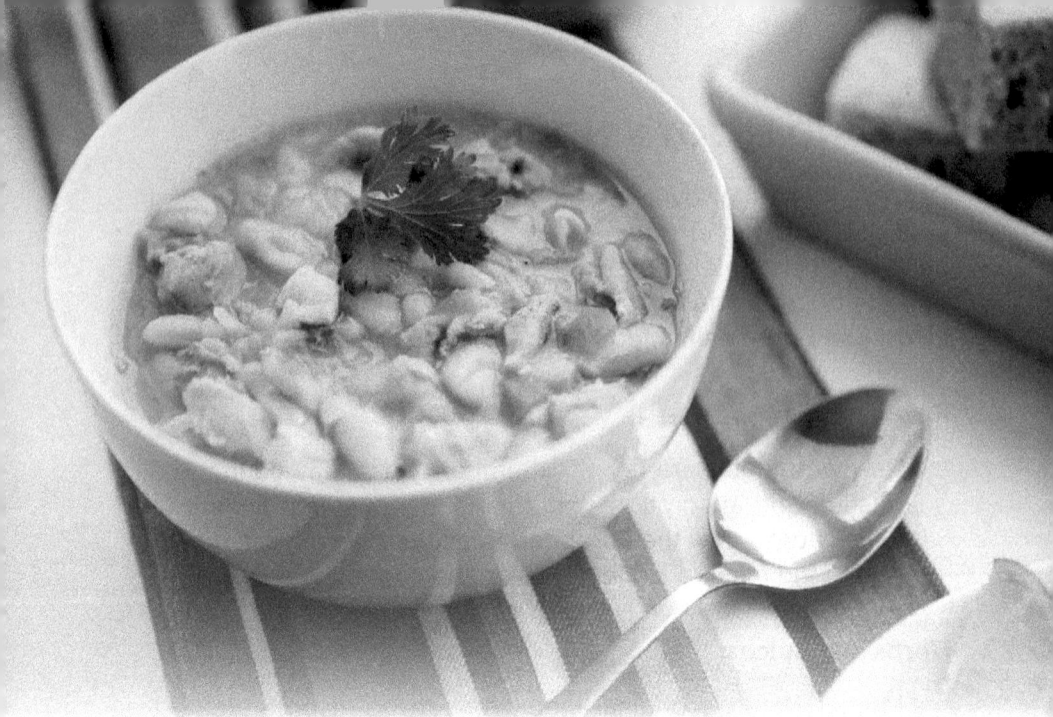

White Chicken Chili

6-8 Servings

INGREDIENTS:

- 4 cups chicken broth, sugar free
- 3 - 15.5-oz. cans white beans, drained and rinsed
- 2 lbs. boneless skinless chicken breasts
- 3 -4-oz. cans diced green chiles (extra can of chiles if you if you like extra kick to your chili)
- 1 medium yellow onion, finely chopped
- 3 cloves garlic, minced
- 2 cups frozen corn
- 1 – 14.5 oz. can diced tomatoes
- 2 teaspoons dried oregano
- 1 ½ teaspoons ground cumin
- 1 teaspoon chili powder
- Salt and Pepper to taste (Optional)
- 1 jalapeño, seeded and minced, plus more for serving

FOR TOPPING:

- Sour cream
- Sliced avocado
- Thinly sliced jalapeño
- Freshly chopped cilantro

PROCESS:

1. Add chicken broth, diced tomatoes, drained beans, chicken, green chiles, onion, garlic, jalapeño, oregano, chili powder and cumin to your slow cooker.
2. Season with salt and pepper and cook on high for 2 to 3 hours, until chicken is tender.
3. Remove chicken from chili and shred. For a thicken chili, use a potato masher to gently mash about 1/3 of the beans before returning chicken to slow cooker.
4. Stir in shredded chicken and corn and cover and season with more salt and pepper if needed.
5. Leave slow cooker on warm until corn heats through and ready to serve.
6. To serve, top with sour cream, avocado, jalapeño, cilantro, and a squeeze of lime juice.

ACTIVITY – EMBRACE AND LOVE MOVEMENT

Yoga and Pilates are ideal activities for all fitness levels, offering numerous benefits such as increased flexibility, strength, and mental clarity. These low-impact exercises can be tailored to individual needs, making them accessible to beginners and challenging for seasoned practitioners.

Yoga offers numerous benefits for both body and mind:

- **Benefits with Breathing:** Focusing on breath control in yoga improves lung capacity, reduces stress, and enhances overall mental clarity and relaxation.
- **Classes:** Attending yoga classes provides structure, professional guidance, and a sense of community, which can enhance your practice.
- **Videos:** Online yoga videos offer flexibility, allowing you to practice at your own pace and convenience, making it easy to fit into your schedule.
- **Chair or Floor:** Yoga can be adapted to your needs, whether it's chair yoga for those with limited mobility, wall yoga or traditional mat-based floor practice.

Pilates strengthens the core and improves overall flexibility and balance:

- **Core Builder:** Pilates focuses on controlled movements that target the core muscles, enhancing stability and strength in the abdominal and lower back areas.
- **Classes:** Joining Pilates classes offers expert supervision, precise instruction, and a motivating environment that can help maximize the benefits of your workout.
- **Videos:** Online Pilates videos provide convenience, allowing you to follow along from home and practice at your own pace.
- **Chair or Floor Versions:** Pilates can be adapted for different needs, with chair or wall versions for those requiring low-impact exercises and traditional mat-based sessions for a comprehensive workout.

Enjoy incorporating these flexible low-impact movement activities.

KINDNESS – CULTIVATE IT IN YOUR DAILY LIFE

Acts of kindness towards animals and their owners are vital for fostering compassion and empathy in our communities. Animals give unconditional love and being a pet owner often means you are often more likely to give and receive unconditional love.

Pet Therapy Visits:

If you have a well-behaved pet, consider becoming part of a therapy animal team. Visit hospitals, nursing homes, or schools to provide comfort to those in need. My younger sister, Anne, in assisted living, feels so much better when a family member brings their dog.

Be Social with Your Pet:

Sharing your pet with others is a wonderful act of kindness. When we took our 3-year-old Mollie to a local outdoor winery, she was pampered like never before. Everyone wanted to interact with her and give her the obligatory belly rubs. Some even asked to take pictures with her and we made new friends that day.

Adopt or Foster:

Provide a loving home for animals in shelters or rescues. Fostering animals in need helps to reduce overcrowding and gives them a better chance at finding permanent homes. When fostering, the only problem is becoming so attached, you do not want to give them up.

Dog Walking:

Offer to walk dogs for elderly or busy neighbors. Regular walks can enhance the dog's health and provide their owners with peace of mind. I have a friend who volunteered to walk dogs and now has a thriving dog-walking business.

Continue to spread kindness in the animal and human world.

Log Today's Activities and Experiences with The SPEAK Method

Use the questions or comments as a guide or write freely expressing your thoughts!

SELF-CARE — List what practices you will implement for your financial security.

_____
_____
_____
_____
_____
_____
_____

PASSION — Write done your first SMART goals for one of your passions.

_____
_____
_____
_____
_____
_____
_____
_____

EAT AND ENJOY — What spices and raw foods are you going to eat?

ACTIVITY — Write down some simple yoga stretches you are going to start with.

KINDNESS – How do you enjoy connecting with animals?

_____
_____
_____
_____
_____

ADDITIONAL NOTES

_____
_____
_____
_____
_____

DAILY REPORT CARD OF LIFE – How did you SPEAK today?

Grade Your Day, no D's or F's Allowed!

    A – Amazing
    B – Better than yesterday
    C – Challenging but working on it

DAY 28

> *"Playing dress-up begins at age five and never truly ends."*
> **Kate Spade**

SELF-CARE – PRACTICE IT DAILY

Do you have fond memories as a child of dress-up games or dress-up day at school? Whether it's for a night out with friends, a solo date or at home by yourself, putting on an outfit that makes you feel amazing can have a positive impact on your mood and confidence.

Dress Up with Friends:

- Dressing up can elevate any social event, making it more enjoyable and memorable. When a group of girlfriends and I went on trips, we typically dressed casually for walks on the beach or strolls through Paris. However, we always chose one night to dress up like queens! It was a fun and unforgettable highlight of every trip.

Dress Up for Solo Date:

- Taking the time to select and wear a thoughtfully chosen outfit can be a mindful practice, helping you to focus on the present moment and your own needs. Years ago, a friend who worked from home had a daily motto: "Get up, dress up, and show up." You are worth the effort and deserve to feel fabulous!

Dress Up to Feel Good:

- If you're feeling stuck in a routine, dressing up can be a fun way to break the monotony.

    Working mostly from home, I found myself in a rut, wearing the same workout clothes or comfy sweats and t-shirts every day. I make it a point to dress up every week, and it has improved my mood, productivity, and interactions with others.

    When you look your best, you feel your best!

PASSION – DISCOVER AND IGNITE IT

A favorite and deeply profound Japanese concept, Ikigai, dates back over a thousand years. In Japanese, "iki," means life, and "gai," means value or worth. This concept is about discovering the harmony between what you love, what you excel at, what the world needs, and what you can be compensated for. I am deeply grateful that my passion for helping people feel youthful and my love of cooking align with my Ikigai. I do what I love, excel at it, provide needed services, and can earn from them.

What You Love:

- Pursue passions that bring you joy and fulfillment. Engaging in activities you love helps cultivate happiness, motivation, and purpose. It will also fuel your spirit, ignite creativity, and create a profound sense of satisfaction and meaning in your life.

What You're Good At:

- Leveraging your skills and strengths is key to success. Excelling in what you're good at builds confidence, enhances performance, and opens doors to new opportunities for growth.

What the World Needs:

- By addressing global needs and current societal challenges, you provide significant value and drive positive change. This will create a legacy, empowering people now and for future generations.

What You Can Be Paid For:

- Turning your talents into income can be challenging, but it is incredibly empowering when achieved. Earning from your expertise brings long-term financial stability, aligns your work with your passion, and validates your professional worth.

Reflecting on these four elements can help you find a fulfilling path.

EAT AND ENJOY – NOURISHING FOOD

Introduce children to nourishing food from a young age to instill healthy eating habits that last a lifetime. Ensure that all family members sit down together for dinner, creating an opportunity to connect and share the day's experiences without the distraction of digital devices.

Involve Children in Cooking:

- Involving them in the cooking process not only imparts valuable skills but also increases their willingness to try new foods. Simple tasks like washing vegetables or stirring ingredients can make meal preparation fun.

Have More "Cans" than "Cannots":

- Focus on positive language around food and highlight the abundance of healthy options they can enjoy. Instead of saying what they can't have, celebrate all the delicious foods they can eat, such as colorful fruits, crunchy vegetables, and whole grains.

Have Food on Hand:

- Keeping a well-stocked pantry and fridge with healthy staples ensures that you can quickly prepare nutritious meals and snacks. Items like fresh fruits, vegetables, whole-grain pasta, lean proteins, and low-fat dairy products make it easier to whip up balanced meals without the stress of last-minute grocery runs.

Create Meals Adults and Kids Will Eat:

- Find a balance between dishes that satisfy both children and adults. Opt for recipes that can be easily adapted to meet everyone's preferences. For example, a taco night can feature a variety of toppings and fillings. Enjoy **Easy Shredded Chicken Tacos** made with rotisserie chicken.

Enjoy making nourishing and engaging meals for the entire family.

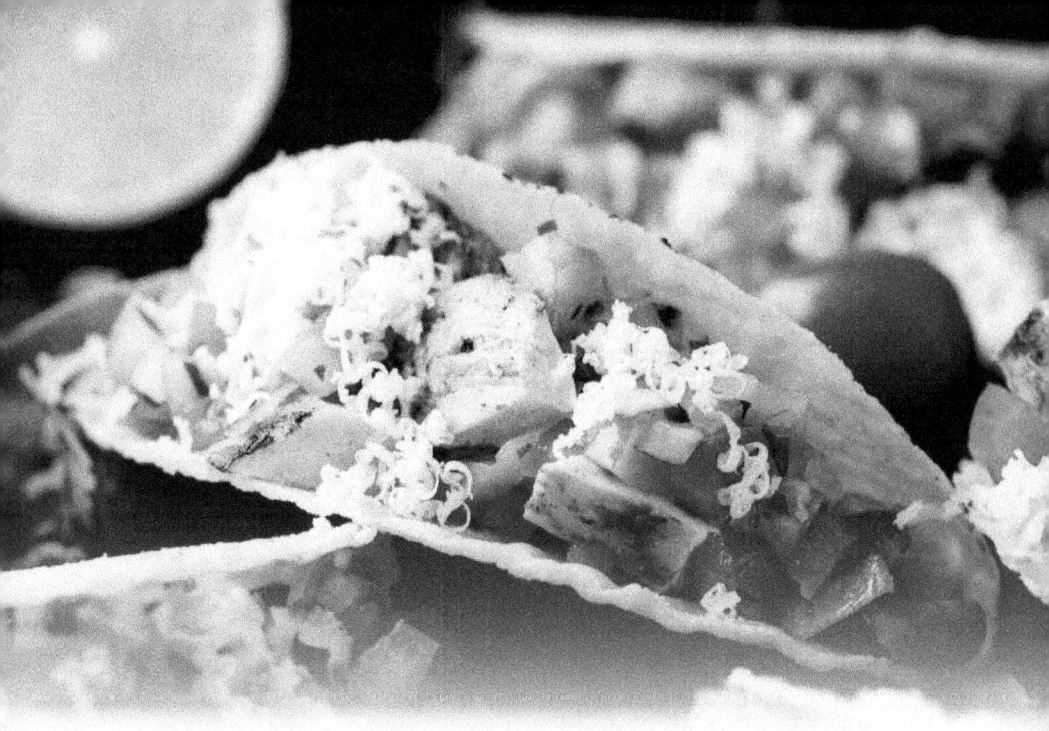

Easy Shredded Chicken Tacos

6 - 8 Servings

INGREDIENTS:

- 1 rotisserie chicken
- 1 teaspoon ground cumin
- 1 Tablespoon chili powder
- 1 teaspoon garlic powder
- 1 teaspoon onion powder
- 1 teaspoon salt
- 1 chopped small yellow onion
- ¼ teaspoon cayenne pepper, optional
- 3/4 cup salsa
- ½ cup chicken stock or bone broth, no sugar added
- 8 corn tortillas
- ¼ cup cilantro, roughly chopped
- ½ cup shredded sharp cheddar

PROCES

1. Debone rotisserie chicken and shred with two forks.

2. Place chicken, onion, salsa, and stock in a large deep skillet.
3. Add cumin, chili powder, garlic powder, onion powder, salt and cayenne if using.
4. Cook on simmer for 10-15 minutes or until liquid evaporates.
5. Serve with warmed corn tortillas.
6. Top with fresh cilantro and shredded sharp cheddar.

ACTIVITY – EMBRACE AND LOVE MOVEMENT

Both canoeing and kayaking provide a full-body workout while allowing you to connect with nature. When I lived in Iowa, I owned a canoe and enjoyed paddling through the rivers of the Midwest and the Boundary Waters of Northern Minnesota. My kayaking experiences include paddling through a cave in Thailand and during a white-water rafting trip in the Grand Canyon. In a calm stretch of water in the canyon, a friend let me try his kayak. Just as I started to get the hang of it, the waters turned rough, and I had to be rescued! The moral of the story: try kayaking for the first time on a calm river or lake.

Where to Do:

- Canoeing and kayaking can be enjoyed on various bodies of water, including lakes, rivers, and even in the ocean. Local parks often have designated areas for these activities.

Basics of How to Do:

- Begin by taking a beginner's course or by sitting in the front of a canoe with an experienced paddler. The person in the back is responsible for steering the boat, allowing the front person to focus on maintaining momentum and enjoying the view.

Muscle Groups Worked:

- A variety of muscle groups are worked including the core muscles for stability and balance. Your arms, shoulders, and back muscles are constantly working with each paddle stroke. Additionally, your legs provide support and assist in maintaining balance, working your lower body indirectly.

Experience nature's tranquility while getting a full-body workout.

KINDNESS – CULTIVATE IT IN YOUR DAILY LIFE

Teaching children kindness is essential for fostering a compassionate and empathetic society. By guiding them in small, everyday actions, we can instill in them a lifelong habit of kindness that extends to all areas of their lives.

Kindness with Friends and Family:

- Encourage children to listen actively to their friends and family members. Teach them to share their toys and belongings, and to express appreciation through words or small gestures.

Kindness with Strangers:

- Demonstrate simple acts of kindness towards strangers, such as holding the door open or helping someone in need. Encourage your child to smile and greet people politely.

Kindness at School:

- Urge children to include other classmates in games and group activities. Teach them to offer help to a peer who might be struggling with schoolwork or feeling left out. Praise them for standing up against bullying and promoting a positive classroom environment.

Kindness in Public Places:

- Show children how to be considerate in public spaces by speaking softly and waiting patiently in lines. Encourage them to say "please" and "thank you" with service workers and respect shared spaces by cleaning up after themselves.

  I recently witnessed a heartwarming scene where two young girls rushed to help an elderly woman who had dropped her purse on the grocery store floor. I made sure to commend their mother for raising such kind children.

Encouraging actions of kindness at a young age will contribute to a more joyous world.

Log Today's Activities and Experiences with The SPEAK Method

Use the questions or comments as a guide or write freely expressing your thoughts!

SELF-CARE – When are you going to dress up for fun?

_____
_____
_____
_____
_____
_____
_____
_____

PASSION – What is your "Ikigai"?

_____
_____
_____
_____
_____
_____
_____
_____

EAT AND ENJOY NOURISHING FOOD – What children can you influence with good food choices?

ACTIVITY – Do you have friends that have a canoe or kayak? Ask them to take you for a paddle or look for local for groups to join.

KINDNESS – List how you will set an example of being kind when around children.

_____
_____
_____
_____
_____
_____

ADDITIONAL NOTES

_____
_____
_____
_____
_____
_____

DAILY REPORT CARD OF LIFE – How did you SPEAK today?

Grade Your Day, no D's or F's Allowed!

- **A** – Amazing
- **B** – Better than yesterday
- **C** – Challenging but working on it

Interview
Michelle Land, BS in Psychology, Master of Science in Management

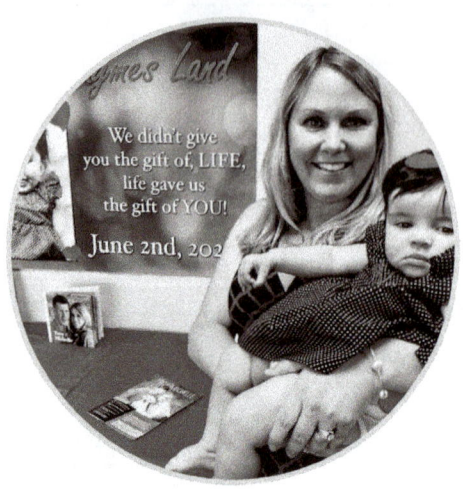

SELF-CARE – PRACTICE IT DAILY

I do little things like go to the Chiropractor every week. It "fills my bucket" to stay connected with my family and friends, even if it is only a quick "hello, how are you?" call. I also allow myself "Veg Out" time snuggling with my dogs while deep breathing or reading my favorite book.

PASSION – DISCOVER AND IGNITE IT

Family in general is my passion. After my husband and I could not have children and spent hundreds of thousands on trying, I concentrated on my career. Also, my husband and I enjoyed traveling and became scuba divers. Then, at the age of 45 we were blessed to adopt a baby girl. My passion to be a mom was finally fulfilled. I make it a point to give her lots of hugs and tell her I love her so many times that she replies "Mom, I know!"

EAT AND ENJOY - NOURISHING FOOD

Instead of going out to eat, we cook most of our food from scratch. I have also taught my four-year-old daughter to make better choices. Instead of saying "no, you cannot have that cookie", I give her a choice "for your snack do you want carrots or cottage cheese?" From a young age she has helped me in the kitchen with her own cooking stand and kid friendly tools.

ACTIVITY – EMBRACE AND LOVE MOVEMENT

For some of my movements, I do intense cleaning, even getting on my hands and knees to scrub floors. I take my dogs for daily walks and when my daughter wants to watch a movie, I say "let's go play outside." We spend time running through the grass and discovering new bugs and flowers. If I do make it to the gym, rather than a treadmill, I enjoy the socialization of classes.

KINDNESS – CULTIVATE IT IN YOUR DAILY LIFE

My parents were the best example of kindness. My very first memory of my dad was him saying "It is ok to not like someone but never hate them." Mom has always shown kindness in her devotion to friends and family. She is the first person to be excited for someone, always sharing her joy. These important lessons are some of the first that I have taught my young daughter.

DAY 29

"We all have heroes. We all look up to people who we think have achieved something miraculous, and in turn, they inspire us to push our boundaries."
Richard Branson

SELF-CARE – PRACTICE IT DAILY

Essential oils are the concentrated essence of a plant, distilled from its leaves, seeds, flowers, roots, or bark. Through the distillation process, the plant's therapeutic properties are captured and transformed into essential oil. Several years ago, I had the opportunity to attend a series of classes taught by an internationally certified aromatherapist. The knowledge I gained was invaluable. Due to their high concentration, use with care and respect.

Purchase therapeutic essential oils and a diffuser from a natural or specialty store. Additionally, obtain a carrier oil, such as coconut or jojoba oil, to dilute the essential oils for safe application on the skin.

Start with Basics:

- Lavender: For a sleep aid, put a few drops on a small cloth inside your pillowcase, rub a drop on each temple, or diffuse it next to your bed. Additionally, lavender is beneficial for healing burns and cuts. I have prevented many cooking burns from blistering, and when mixed with aloe, it has soothed my skin after unexpected sunburns, helping to prevent peeling.
- Rosemary: Enhances mental clarity. When tackling a big project or needing to focus, diffuse it near your desk. Place a couple of drops in the palm of your hand, rub them together, and cup your hands over your nose and mouth while breathing in deeply.
- Peppermint: Beneficial for headaches, digestive support, and boosting energy. For energy, add a drop to your water or rub it on the back of your neck to alleviate tension headaches.

Enjoy the benefits of Mother Nature's Medicine!

PASSION – DISCOVER AND IGNITE IT

Reflect on the individuals you admire, be they real or fictional, and identify the attributes that resonate with you. Often, the qualities you appreciate in them are those you aspire to embody. Use these insights to discover and ignite your passion.

Personal Mentors:

- Individuals who have directly guided, supported, and inspired you in your life, such as family members, teachers, or coaches. My mother was my first personal hero. When she married my Navy father, she left her large family in Massachusetts to move to the unfamiliar plains of Iowa, where she knew almost no one. Her resilience was matched by her incredible kindness, as she willingly took in neighborhood children and friends' kids during times of need. May I continue to exemplify these traits.

Historical Figures:

- Influential people from history whose achievements and legacy have left a lasting impact, like Martin Luther King Jr., Marie Curie, or Mahatma Gandhi. Choose an individual or individuals whose legacy resonates with yours.

Industry Leaders:

- Seek out professionals who have made notable contributions to your field of interest, such as innovators, entrepreneurs, or thought leaders. Identify a leader in your area of passion and read any articles or books they have authored.

Everyday Heroes:

- Who are the ordinary individuals you admire for performing extraordinary acts of kindness and bravery in daily life, often without recognition? What actions do they take that align with your passions?

Discovering more about the people you admire can be both enjoyable and insightful.

EAT AND ENJOY – NOURISHING FOOD

The decision to adopt a gluten-free diet can be motivated by various reasons, from managing celiac disease to reducing gluten sensitivity, or simply seeking to improve overall wellness by limiting wheat consumption. Eating gluten-free can seem challenging at first, but with the right strategies, it will become a seamless part of your daily routine.

Read Labels Carefully:

- Always check food labels for hidden sources of gluten. Ingredients like wheat, barley, and rye are obvious, but gluten can also be found in less apparent additives such as malt, modified food starch, and certain flavorings.

Focus on Naturally Gluten-Free Foods:

- Base your diet around whole foods that are naturally free from gluten, such as fruits, vegetables, lean meats, fish, eggs, dairy, nuts, and seeds. Grains like rice, quinoa, and corn are excellent gluten-free options.

Experiment with Gluten-Free Cooking and Baking:

- Invest in gluten-free flour: almond flour, coconut flour, and gluten-free blends can be used to create delicious baked goods. Bake these tasty **Praline Pecan Pumpkin Bars.**

Choose Organic:

- Glyphosate is a chemical compound used primarily to kill weeds, but it can also be applied as a desiccant to dry out crops like wheat. A client experienced adverse reactions, such as bloating and gas, to bread in the U.S. However, when she visited Europe and ate bread from local bakeries, she did not experience the same adverse reactions.

The wide availability of gluten-free foods makes it much easier, and many stores have a gluten-free section.

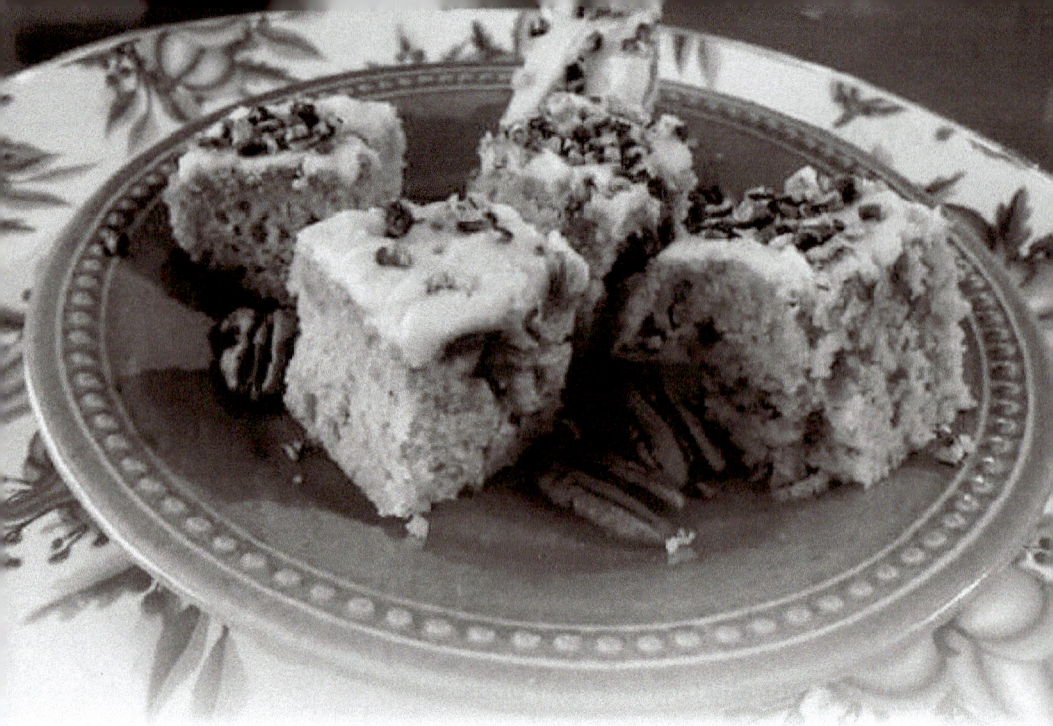

Praline Pecan Pumpkin Bars

12-15 Servings

CAKE INGREDIENTS:

- 2 cups white whole wheat or gluten free flour
- 1 teaspoon baking powder
- 1/2 teaspoon baking soda
- 1 teaspoon ground cinnamon
- 1 teaspoon ground ginger
- 1/2 teaspoon ground nutmeg
- 1/2 teaspoon sea salt
- 1 15 oz can pumpkin puree
- 3/4 cup granulated monk fruit
- 1 cup avocado oil
- 4 eggs

FROSTING INGREDIENTS:

- 2 1/2 cups powdered monk fruit
- 3/4 cup pure coconut sugar
- 6 Tablespoons unsalted butter
- 1/3 cup heavy cream
- 1 teaspoon vanilla extract
- 1 cup toasted chopped pecans

CAKE PROCESS:

1. Preheat oven to 350°F
2. Coat a 13 "x 9 " baking pan with oil spray.
3. Whisk together in a medium bowl flour, baking powder and soda, cinnamon, ginger, nutmeg and salt.
4. In a large bowl, whisk together pumpkin, monk fruit. oil and eggs until smooth.
5. Add flour mixture to pumpkin mixture and whisk just until incorporated.
6. Pour mixture into prepared baking pan and smooth top. Bake in preheated oven for about 25 minutes until cake is springy and toothpick inserted into center comes out clean.
7. Transfer to a wire rack and allow to cool for about 1 hour.

FROSTING PROCESS:

1. Sift monk fruit powder in a large heat proof bowl and set aside.
2. Bring coconut sugar, butter and cream to a light boil for 1 minute. Immediately pour cream mixture into bowl with powdered sugar.
3. Add vanilla and whisk vigorously until mixture is smooth.
4. Working quickly, spread frosting over cooled cake. (Frosting will harden quickly)
5. Top with chopped pecans. Let sit for about 30 minutes before serving.

Store in covered container for 3 days at room temperature or in fridge for about 7 days.

ACTIVITY – EMBRACE AND LOVE MOVEMENT

I'll admit from the beginning: I am not a golfer! To me, chasing a ball for hours can be quite frustrating. However, golf courses are often beautiful and provide an opportunity to enjoy nature. My husband, on the other hand, has been an avid golfer his entire life, attending college with a golf scholarship. I enjoy being his cart girl! Even if you use a cart, there are plenty of opportunities to get a good amount of walking.

Warm-Up and Cool Down with Stretching:

- Start your round with a vigorous warm-up, including stretches and light cardio like brisk walking. After your round, do a full body stretch to improve flexibility and aid recovery.

Speed Up Your Pace Between Shots:

- Increase your walking speed between holes or shots. A brisk pace can turn your round of golf into a light cardio session, helping you burn more calories.

Engage in Core Exercises While Waiting:

- While waiting for others to take their shots, use the time to do standing core exercises like side bends, twists, or leg lifts to strengthen your core muscles.

Not a Golfer? Attend a Tournament:

- Attending a tournament often involves walking several miles throughout the day. During our time in Arizona, we attended the Phoenix Open, a professional golf tournament that involved a lot of walking under the hot desert sun and concluded with music and a lively dance party.

Give golf a try, you may be surprised at how much movement it involves.

KINDNESS – CULTIVATE IT IN YOUR DAILY LIFE

Mentoring or tutoring someone in a skill or subject you excel in, whether in person or online, is a profound act of kindness that empowers others, boosts their confidence, and fosters a supportive community of learning and growth. I absolutely love teaching cooking classes online or at the beloved Hendersonville, NC shop, Homemade Pasta Noodles. Sharing my favorite recipes during their "Lunch and Learn" or guest chef series is a joy. I enjoy the engaging conversations, questions, and interactions that happen before, during and after each class. Reach out to your local library, community center, schools, shops, or YMCA to volunteer your expertise.

Academic Tutoring:

- Offer one-on-one or group sessions in subjects like math, science, or language arts to help students improve their understanding, boost their confidence, and enhance their academic performance in school.

Career Guidance:

- Provide advice and support for individuals looking to advance in their careers, including resume building, interview practice, networking strategies, and gaining industry-specific skills through continuous learning and professional development courses.

Life Skills Coaching:

- Teach essential life skills such as time management, financial planning, or effective communication to help individuals navigate everyday challenges, increase their productivity, and enhance their personal and professional relationships, ultimately improving their overall quality of life.

Healthy Living Mentorship:

- Share your knowledge on topics such as nutrition, exercise, mental wellness, stress management techniques, and mindfulness practices to guide others in achieving healthier and more balanced lifestyles.

Make your classes or mentorship meetings fun and exciting.

Log Today's Activities and Experiences with The SPEAK Method

Use the questions or comments as a guide or write freely expressing your thoughts!

SELF-CARE – What are your favorite scents to try in an essential oil?

_____
_____
_____
_____
_____
_____
_____

PASSION – List individuals you admire.

_____
_____
_____
_____
_____
_____
_____

EAT AND ENJOY NOURISHING FOOD – What are some gluten-free foods you have tried and enjoyed?

ACTIVITY – When was the last time you were on a golf course? What did you enjoy about it?

KINDNESS – List skills that you have to offer through a class or one-on-one mentorship. Make a list of people or places to teach or mentor.

ADDITIONAL NOTES

DAILY REPORT CARD OF LIFE – How did you SPEAK today?

Grade Your Day, no D's or F's Allowed!

- **A** – Amazing
- **B** – Better than yesterday
- **C** – Challenging but working on it

DAY 30

> "What we have once enjoyed we can never lose. All that we love deeply becomes a part of us."
> **Helen Keller**

Congratulations on reaching Day 30! By embracing The SPEAK Method, you've taken the first steps toward feeling youthful at any age. Keep going strong, you deserve it!

SELF-CARE – PRACTICE IT DAILY

- I thoroughly enjoyed participating in these self-care activities and hope you did as well. Remember, self-care is an ongoing journey. Reflect on what you've learned, celebrate your progress, and continue to listen to the needs of your body and mind. As my friend Cody's grandmother said, "Full throttle to the grave." Give it all you got!

PASSION – DISCOVER AND IGNITE IT

- Being part of this journey of discovering and igniting passion with you has been truly enlightening, and I hope you have found it equally inspiring. May your progress and enthusiasm continue and be incredibly fulfilling.

EAT AND ENJOY – NOURISHING FOOD

- My passion for cooking, sharing new recipes, and offering cooking tips was extremely energizing. It brought me joy to create nourishing meals that every member of your family will enjoy. Keep experimenting with new ideas and always remember to enjoy your time in the kitchen!

ACTIVITY – EMBRACE AND LOVE MOVEMENT

- Writing this book has encouraged me to "practice what I preach" and incorporate movement into my day. Exercise does not have to be a "bad eight letter word," make it fun, enjoyable, and sustainable.
- My neighbor Dave recently shared what a good friend said to him, "Davey, if you stop you die." A great motto to live by.

KINDNESS – CULTIVATE IT IN YOUR DAILY LIFE

- Through this journey, I've come to realize that kindness is the cornerstone of The SPEAK Method. My wise 85-year-old neighbor Anne put it perfectly: "Kindness is the most important thing to have in your life—why be ugly and mean when you can be kind?"

Let's work together to create a kind and joyful world.
In Gratitude and Appreciation,

Kathy

Share the Lessons and Experiences You've Gained Using The SPEAK Method

SELF-CARE – PRACTICE IT DAILY

_____
_____
_____
_____
_____
_____
_____

PASSION – DISCOVER AND IGNITE IT

_____
_____
_____
_____
_____
_____
_____
_____

EAT AND ENJOY – NOURISHING FOOD

ACTIVITY – EMBRACE AND LOVE MOVEMENT

KINDNESS – CULTIVATE IT IN YOUR DAILY LIFE

_____
_____
_____
_____
_____
_____

ADDITIONAL NOTES

_____
_____
_____
_____
_____
_____
_____

FINAL 30-DAY REPORT CARD OF LIFE WITH The SPEAK Method

Grade Your 30-Day Progress, no D's or F's Allowed!

- **A** – Amazing
- **B** – Better than yesterday
- **C** – Challenging but working on it

Author Note

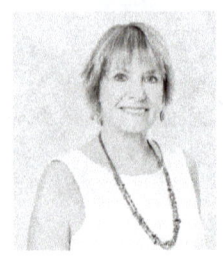

You are holding in your hands the culmination of 40 years of ideas, practices, recipes and knowledge that have lived within my heart and mind. My journey began in the Midwest during the 1950's, where life was simple, and community connections were strong. We played hopscotch and dodgeball on quiet streets, and my first entrepreneurial endeavor was a lemonade stand for local road workers, earning me $50, feeling like the richest person in town!

Though I longed to attend the "big" public school, I attended a small Catholic school and graduated high school with a class of just 99 students. My college years took me to an all-girls school and then to the University of Iowa, where I earned my degree in Bioscience and worked in a microbiology lab.

My love for cooking and entrepreneurial spirit led me to launch Iowa's first organic fine dining restaurant, pioneering local, healthy, and sustainable eating. That same spirit, combined with a passion for skiing, took my husband and me to the Colorado Mountains, where we purchased and expanded a natural foods store and became top wedding caterers in Summit County.

Our journey next took us to an organic coffee farm in Panama, immersing us in local culture and the unique flavors of the tropical rainforest.

Furthering my commitment to wellness, I became a consultant for various nutritional companies, focusing on training and product education.

Now residing in the North Carolina mountains with my husband Harvey and our Westie dog, Mollie Mae, I work as a health coach, personal chef, cooking class instructor and product developer. This allows me to fulfill my passion for helping people through personalized wellness guidance, motivation, and nutritious meals.

Building on my science background and four decades of experience in natural health, I am currently developing a unique liquid whole-plant nutritional product.

www.beyoungernextmonth.com

www.ingramcontent.com/pod-product-compliance
Lightning Source LLC
Chambersburg PA
CBHW060946050426
42337CB00052B/1541